Telehealth and Telemedicine - The Far-Reaching Medicine for Everyone and Everywhere

Edited by Tang-Chuan Wang

Published in London, United Kingdom

Telehealth and Telemedicine - The Far-Reaching Medicine for Everyone and Everywhere
http://dx.doi.org/10.5772/intechopen.100663
Edited by Tang-Chuan Wang

Contributors
Rene Ivan Gonzalez-Fernandez, Margarita Mulet-Cartaya, Gisela Montes de Oca-Colina, Jose Luis Hernandez-Caceres, Jorge Aguilera-Perez, Juan Dayron Lopez-Cardona, Maria Cecilia Vega-Corredor, Alison Watkins, Simon Hoermann, Melanie Tomintz, Somprakas Basu, Sudhir Kumar Singh, Navin Kumar, Farhanul Huda, Jyoti Sharma, Lokavarapu Manoj Joshua, Intan Sabrina Mohamad, Irma Ruslina Defi, András Fittler, Márton Fittler, Róbert György Vida, Xiaoni Zhang, Haoqiang Jiang, Gary Ozanich, Idar Mappangara, Andriany Qanitha, Oseghale Igene, Aimee Ferguson, Lua Perimal-Lewis, Patricia A.H. Williams, Ginger Mudd, Gihan Gunasekara

First published in London, United Kingdom, 2023 by IntechOpen
IntechOpen is the global imprint of INTECHOPEN LIMITED, registered in England and Wales, registration number: 11086078, 5 Princes Gate Court, London, SW7 2QJ, United Kingdom

British Library Cataloguing-in-Publication Data
A catalogue record for this book is available from the British Library

Additional hard and PDF copies can be obtained from orders@intechopen.com

Telehealth and Telemedicine - The Far-Reaching Medicine for Everyone and Everywhere Edited by Tang-Chuan Wang
p. cm.

This title is part of the Biomedical Engineering Book Series, Volume 16
Topic: Bioinformatics and Medical Informatics
Series Editor: Robert Koprowski
Topic Editor: Slawomir Wilczynski

Print ISBN 978-1-80356-194-3
Online ISBN 978-1-80356-195-0
eBook (PDF) ISBN 978-1-80356-196-7
ISSN 2631-5343

IntechOpen Book Series

Biomedical Engineering

Volume 16

Aims and Scope of the Series

Biomedical Engineering is one of the fastest-growing interdisciplinary branches of science and industry. The combination of electronics and computer science with biology and medicine has improved patient diagnosis, reduced rehabilitation time, and helped to facilitate a better quality of life. Nowadays, all medical imaging devices, medical instruments, or new laboratory techniques result from the cooperation of specialists in various fields. The series of Biomedical Engineering books covers such areas of knowledge as chemistry, physics, electronics, medicine, and biology. This series is intended for doctors, engineers, and scientists involved in biomedical engineering or those wanting to start working in this field.

Meet the Series Editor

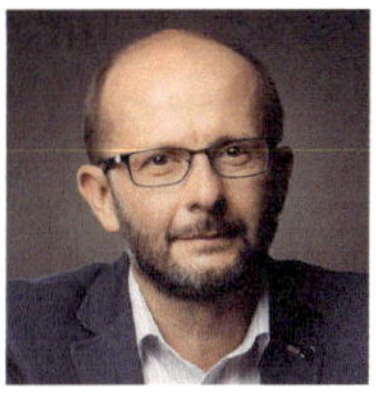

Robert Koprowski, MD (1997), Ph.D. (2003), Habilitation (2015), is an employee of the University of Silesia, Poland, Institute of Computer Science, Department of Biomedical Computer Systems. For 20 years, he has studied the analysis and processing of biomedical images, emphasizing the full automation of measurement for a large inter-individual variability of patients. Dr. Koprowski has authored more than a hundred research papers with dozens in impact factor (IF) journals and has authored or co-authored six books. Additionally, he is the author of several national and international patents in the field of biomedical devices and imaging. Since 2011, he has been a reviewer of grants and projects (including EU projects) in biomedical engineering.

Meet the Volume Editor

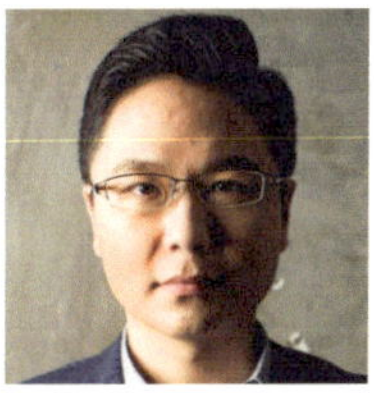

Dr. Tang-Chuan Wang is an otolaryngologist (head and neck surgeon) in Taiwan. He is also a research scholar at Harvard Medical School and the University of Iowa Hospital. During his career, he has worked at Stanford University, the University of Pennsylvania, Boston Children's Hospital and Massachusetts Eye and Ear. In addition to his clinical work, in recent years he has branched out into public health in Taiwan, with a focus on innovation and telemedicine. He always says that "in theoretical or practical aspects, no innovation is a backward step". As a result of his contribution to biodesign, he was invited to join the Executive Committee of Taiwan's Advanced Joint R & D Center.

Contents

Preface

Telehealth allows clinicians to care for patients at a distance via electronic information technologies. The term covers clinical and non-clinical services, including monitoring, diagnosis, and treatment, as well as delivery of preventative care and health promotion. Telemedicine is a more common term which describes remote clinical services.

The major impact of COVID-19 has caused telemedicine to become mainstream since the end of 2019. Clinicians are having to use tele-consultation, tele-monitoring, tele-pharmacy, tele-rehabilitation, tele-surgery and other remote methods and technologies to assess and treat patients. We now have an opportunity to re-assess whether existing telemedicine is sufficient to meet higher-level medical needs in theory and practice.

The patient-centric model of care means that information and interaction originate from the patient. Personalized data generated by various monitoring technologies are jointly managed by patients and medical staff. Medical staff will supervise artificial intelligence (AI) algorithms to understand the patient's specific condition and provide the best decision-making and treatment, moving us ever closer to the ideal of precision medicine.

This book incorporates new developments as well as future prospects in the ever-expanding field of telehealth and telemedicine. It will be a resource for medical staff (physicians, surgeons, family doctors, ENT doctors, audiologists, psychologists, registered nurses, technologists), specialists in sleep medicine, social workers, public health practitioners, researchers in basic medicine, experts in science, students, and even patients themselves.

I would like to thank all the authors who have dedicated their time and expertise to this book, as well as everyone who has contributed to the editorial process, including the author service manager, the publishing process manager, the commissioning editor, and the technical editor. Their efforts have resulted in a successful academic work. Finally, I am grateful as ever to everyone who has been part of my own journey, including my family, teachers and colleagues.

Tang-Chuan Wang (Vincent Wang)
Chairman of Otolaryngology-Head and Neck Surgery,
China Medical University Hsinchu Hospital,
Taiwan

School of Medicine,
College of Medicine,
China Medical University,
Taiwan

Department of Biomedical Engineering,
College of Biomedical Engineering,
China Medical University,
Taiwan

Research Scholar of Harvard Medical School,
MA, USA

Research Scholar of University of Iowa Hospitals and Clinics,
IA, USA

Member of American Academy of Otolaryngology-Head and Neck Surgery

Fellow of the American College of Surgeons

Section 1

The Far-Reaching Telehealth and Telemedicine on Health Education, Consultation and Monitoring

Chapter 1

Design Insights to Support the Development of Effective Virtual Reality Nicotine and Vaping Dependency Therapy Scenarios for Future Telehealth

Maria Cecilia Vega-Corredor, Simon Hoermann, Alison Watkins and Melanie Tomintz

Abstract

Vaping, or the use of electronic nicotine delivery systems (ENDS), has grown rapidly worldwide and is becoming an epidemic among youth in many countries. Invented as a method to help to quit smoking, ENDS are very popular, reaching increasing numbers of users and becoming a health concern. Virtual reality technology (VRT) represents an important tool for conducting addiction-associated interventions, including telemedicine. The design and quality of virtual reality scenarios (VRS) used for VR interventions are fundamental. How well VRS can replicate real-world scenarios has an impact on how realistic the VR immersion experiences are. Thus, VRS development influences therapeutic outcomes. VRT is used for interventions and treatments for smoking-related nicotine addiction but has yet to be validated for vaping-related disorders. Since vaping represents a technological step forward in nicotine consumption, the accurate contextualization of environments surrounding vapers is fundamental for developing advanced VR tools for the prevention and treatment of vaping disorders. Here, we present the results of focus group discussion with young vapers in New Zealand. The knowledge gained from this study will be used to design VRS for cue exposure and reactivity as a first step toward developing effective solutions for vaping disorders using VR interventions and telemedicine.

Keywords: virtual reality (VR), electronic nicotine delivery systems (ENDS), vaping, nicotine dependence, interventions, VR in telemedicine

1. Introduction

Vaping, which refers to the use of electronic nicotine delivery systems (ENDS, e-cigarettes, vapes, or nicotine vaping devices), has grown rapidly worldwide [1, 2], and is currently considered to be an epidemic among teens and young adults in countries, such as the United States [3]. From an initial cig-a-like device, developed to help to quit smoking, ENDS evolved rapidly into a wide spectrum of gadgets that are used either as tobacco cigarette replacements or for recreational purposes, transforming vaping into a paradigm of its own. Despite being relatively new, ENDS have been subjected to extensive study, with research topics ranging from vaping demographics to their latest technological developments. Nonetheless, as the number of vapers grows, many gaps exist in what is known about vaping, especially in fundamental issues such as those related to long-term health effects [4] and addiction. However, vaping has been shown to be a multifactorial practice that not only relates to a physiological need for nicotine but also responds to different cultural, socio-economic, and psychological aspects that are yet to be fully understood. In order to characterize vaping contexts, some consumers' features, such as ENDS or smoking habit (tobacco cigarettes, hookah, or waterpipe tobacco), use history and status may be of help by providing some evidence in the effort to achieve a better understanding of this trend. Thus, vaper status, such as if they are ex-smokers, dual users, or vape only, has been identified [5]. According to the user status, the context surrounding vaping, preferences, habits, and behavior may change. Therefore, the approach to study vaping-related problems should be adjusted accordingly.

Aside from conventional methods used in interventions and treatment of behavioral and health disorders, virtual reality technology (VRT) represents a reliable and more personalized technique that can be used under well-developed and lifelike controllable settings [6]. VRT has already been used satisfactorily for craving assessments, cue exposure, and cue reactivity therapy for smoking-associated interventions and treatments [7]. As vaping is associated with smoking and mainly with nicotine use, VRT may be suitable for the study of vaping-related disorders. Nevertheless, a key factor in the implementation of VRT for the study of behavioral and substance use disorders depends on how well real-life situations, locations, and features associated with the targeted condition are identified and characterized. Realistic representations are fundamental to inform the development of virtual reality scenarios (VRS) in which the VR studies take place. These technical systems provide a 3D vision, 360-degree range, and head tracking where the recreated real-life situations are presented [8]. The design and technical development of the VRS will determine how inclusive, extensive, and vivid the resemblances that the system generates are. Thus, it determines how good the VR immersion experience can be and influences the perceptions and reactions experienced by each patient. Recently VR and telehealth have effectively been used to provide different types of interventions, which not only can help improve health conditions but also enable social connectedness and psychological support. For many, in-person consultations may be difficult and costly. VR in telehealth allows the interactive use of online scenarios that represent a cost-effective solution for those who need treatment but for some reason are unable to visit their therapist or doctor's office [9].

As vaping is relatively new but growing at a rapid rate, the situations, locations, and reasons why people vape may be dynamic and changing according to time and geographical location. In New Zealand (NZ), nicotine e-liquids started being sold legally in 2018 [10]. Since then, the country's policies have been changing, and more recently, additional regulations toward vaping products have been put in place [11]. In recent years, NZ has experienced a sharp increase in ENDS use, mostly in teens [12]. In parallel, tobacco cigarette taxes were increased under a plan to achieve a smoke-free country by 2025. This plan included campaigns to switch to vaping as a way to stop smoking tobacco cigarettes [13]. As ENDS evolved rapidly, vaping represents a technological step forward into a new way of nicotine use and dependence [14], which although presented as a less harmful and disruptive way to use nicotine, may signify an underlying cause of long-term health issues. Understanding and accurately characterizing the environments and contexts in which people vape, and the reasons why is fundamental for developing strategies and advanced aid tools in the current and future health issues associated with vaping.

This qualitative study was part of a wider project that aimed to develop and test VRS associated with vaping. The aim of this study was to perform focus group discussions to inform our research about real environments where young people vape in NZ. Thus, we interviewed a diverse sample of university students who had experimented with ENDS, to learn about their vaping experiences. The final VRS will be used for the study of vaping cue exposure and reactivity in VR and telehealth interventions and treatments.

2. Methods

Focus group discussions were conducted to gain knowledge directly from young adults about their motivations, habits, behavior, contexts, and views associated with vaping. Grounded theory was used as the conceptual research approach [15] since at the time of the study, vaping characteristics and contexts in NZ were not fully identified and a better understanding of the concepts surrounding this practice was necessary to inform the development of realistic vaping VRS. Four focus group sessions were conducted from September to November 2019 at the University of Canterbury (UC - Christchurch, NZ). Recruitment of participants was conducted via an advertisement on UC's social media, TV media, and an event management website. The theoretical sampling method [15], a qualitative method for data collection based on obtaining concepts from data, was used to gain insights into NZ's vaping contexts. We recruited university students that have previously used ENDS.

2.1 Recruitment

Inclusion criteria: being 18+ years having vaped in the past or at the study's time.

Exclusion criteria: having addictions different from smoking or vaping, suffering from mental illness, being associated with a vaping company, and using other nicotine replacement products (nicotine patches, chewing gum, or lozenges). At first contact, all prospective candidates were informed about the project and the focus group aims and checked for inclusion and exclusion criteria.

2.2 Participants

Nine students were selected to participate in the focus group discussions, from whom 7 were males (M) and 2 females (F). The groups composition was: group 1: n = 3 (M); group 2: n = 3 (1F, 2 M); group 3: n = 1 (M); group 4: n = 2 (1F, 1 M). The groups were not arranged by any specific participant characteristics related to vaping habits or views.

2.3 Focus groups procedure

All sessions were scheduled to last up to 2 hours. Before each session, consent forms and questionnaires regarding demographics were distributed and completed by all participants. At the beginning of each session, the moderator gave an introduction, informing each group about the project aim and explaining the focus group objectives, procedures, and ground rules. Verbal consent was requested for video and audio recording. Additionally, participants were assured of anonymity and data confidentiality. Everyone chooses a nickname to be addressed during the discussions. All participants were informed that nicknames will be replaced by codes during the transcription process. The raw recorded data can only be used as material for publications related to the research project.

While any assumptions about users' views, experiences, and behavior associated with vaping were not pre-established, semi-structured interviews [16] were conducted throughout the focus group sessions. Thus, with the aim to cover the study's objectives, an interview guide was developed. Four main topics were considered: background, current context, triggers, and reactions. For each topic, questions were elaborated, aiming to prompt each participant to provide open, free, and in-depth answers. The semi-structured interview scheme helped to steer the discussions while allowing for flexibility [16]. Questions were not necessarily asked in the same order and the moderator was free to follow digressions or asked for clarification if required. Probes were used in some questions to facilitate the process. All participants were free to give any personal opinions. At the end of each session, a small financial token was given to the participants to compensate them for their time. The UC Human Ethics Committee approved this study.

2.4 Transcriptions and coding

All focus group interviews were transcribed into text documents and coded using NVIVO software. At first, using the interview guide, all participants' answers were grouped by related questions. Next, codes were created by finding and grouping similar responses, as well as individual/uniquely relevant answers. Once the data search was exhausted and all possible codes were defined, codes were grouped by theme/topic.

3. Results

3.1 Demographics

The total number of participants was nine (2F and 7 M). The mean age was 24 years; hence, most participants were considered as young adults, from which four were New Zealanders, four Indians, and one German. All participants were students at UC (3 undergraduate and 6 postgraduate) (**Table 1**).

3.2 Participants' vaping profile

In this study, for data analysis, all participants were classified according to their vaping profile:

- *Smoking and vaping habits*: tobacco and e-cigarettes, hookah, and ENDS.
- *Status*: dual user, ENDS (only), and hookah.
- *Current use*: active and inactive; and

Participants code*	Gender	Age group	Country of birth	Educational level	Current occupation	Time in NZ (years)
FG1M1	M	40–44	NZ	Undergraduate	Postgraduate student	>10
FG1M2	M	21–24	Germany	Postgraduate	Postgraduate student	<1
FG1M3	M	18–20	NZ	Secondary	Undergraduate student	>10
FG2M1	M	18–20	NZ	Secondary	Undergraduate student	>10
FG3F1	F	25–29	India	Undergraduate	Postgraduate student	<1
FG3M1	M	21–25	India	Undergraduate	Postgraduate student	<1
FG3M2	M	21–24	India	Undergraduate	Postgraduate student	<1
FG4F1	F	21–24	India	Undergraduate	Postgraduate student	<1
FG4M1	M	18–20	NZ	Secondary	Undergraduate student	>10

**The participants' nicknames were replaced by codes.*

Table 1.
Demographics of ENDS users who participate in vaping focus group discussions (UC, Christchurch NZ, 2019).

- *Current frequency of use*: frequent (few times per week/daily), occasional (sometimes per month), and rare. Thus, according to the habit type, there were five dual users (tobacco and e-cigarettes), two ENDS users only and two hookah users. One of the dual users (FG1M1) presented himself as a predominantly tobacco cigarette smoker (occasional e-cigarette user), and one hookah user (FG3M1) stated that he rarely used tobacco cigarettes, therefore, he was classified as a hookah user (**Table 2**).

3.3 Background: length of use, vaping factors associated with start and continuing vaping

The earliest and latest first use of ENDS by participants were reported around 2009 (FG1M1) and 2018 (FG2M1). Reasons to start vaping were not necessarily associated with one aspect only. Instead, they were a combination of different factors, for six participants the financial aspect was the main reason to start vaping. All five dual users associated high prices of tobacco cigarettes and how ENDS prices help them save money. Other main reasons were: ENDS are more socially acceptable (4 participants), peer pressure (3 participants), and out of curiosity (2 participants). Moreover, only two dual users mentioned quitting smoking as an additional reason to start vaping and one dual user mentioned the need to reduce the intake of tobacco cigarettes. In particular, one participant mentioned a personal relationship: *"I wanted to switch because my girlfriend was like really piss off at me smoking and then so it didn't*

Code	Habits	User status	Current use	Frequency of use
FG1M1	Tobacco cigarettes	Dual	Active	Frequent
	ENDS		Active	Occasional
FG1M2	Tobacco cigarettes	Dual	Active	Occasional
	ENDS		Active	Frequent
FG1M3	Tobacco cigarettes	Dual	Inactive	Frequent (in the past)
	ENDS		Active	Frequent
FG2M1	ENDS	ENDS	Active	Occasional
FG3F1	Tobacco cigarettes	Dual	Inactive	Occasional
	ENDS		Inactive	Occasional
FG3M1	Hookah*	Hookah	Inactive	Occasional
	Tobacco Cigarettes		Active	Occasional
FG3M2	Hookah	Hookah	Inactive	Frequent (in the past)
FG4F1	ENDS	ENDS	Inactive	Rare (in the past)
FG4M1	ENDS	Dual	Active	Frequent
	Tobacco cigarettes		Active	Frequent

**Hookah classification was based on the mechanism to heat and deliver the tobacco smoke used by the hookah, in which the tobacco is heated with charcoal and the smoke is cooled by passing it through water.*

Table 2.
Code and classification of ENDS users who participated in vaping focus group discussions (UC, Christchurch NZ, 2019).

really come from me" (FG1M2). Another mentioned the technological convenience of it, and smell: "*The fact that you don't have to carry a lighter where you go, it seems like a technology advance which was interesting [...] smells good*" (FG3F1). Only one participant mentioned health as an important reason to start vaping. Among dual users, three participants experienced an intermittent pattern of ENDS use, for example, "*Yeah, so I probably have been vaping for about 263 days but, before that, I had probably vaped half a year before and then stopped after a party sort of went out of track. [I] started smoking cigarettes with friends and then sort of went back to rolling cigarettes for about 3–4 months and just went back to vaping because I've had a bit of breakdown about it. I don't want to be wasting money and the fact that I had a lot at stake...*" (FG1M3). In relation to factors associated with continuing vaping, after the initial onset, these included: nicotine (3 dual users), flavor (2 hookah users and 1 dual user), hanging out with friends or socializing (2), convenience and enjoyment (1 dual user): "*It's more convenient than sitting down to have a cigarette because you can vape in the car [...] without like, stinking like tobacco smoke, so that's probably the main reason why I'm still using [...]. Like it's fun so I mean I use it for enjoyment*" (FG4M1). In addition, two participants had already stopped vaping.

3.4 Vaping context: frequency of vaping (currently or at the time of ENDS use), e-liquids preferences, nicotine awareness and relevance, devices used, and common places where participants vape

In general, the participants did not manifest having clear patterns of vaping, their use seemed to be irregular and related to their personal needs or convenience. Keeping this in mind, at the time of the discussions, four participants considered their ENDS use as frequent (3 active and 1 stopped), three occasional, two rare, and two had stopped vaping (**Table 2**). In relation to e-liquid preferences, fruit flavors were the most popular (4 participants). Strawberry, apple, grape, watermelon, and guava were the most commonly used. Three persons indicated menthol and mint as their favorites. For hookah users, bay leaves, and "chilly ice" flavors were preferred. Tobacco flavor was not chosen by anyone, for example, "*I have tried it, like I don't like the tobacco flavor, I like the taste of tobacco I don't like the taste of tobacco vape*" (FG4M1). "*I tried tobacco [vape] [I] absolutely hated it [...], smells like tobacco but it doesn't taste like tobacco, not sure at all*" (FG1M2). In addition, for one dual user fruit flavors have helped him to reduce smoking tobacco cigarettes: "*... I changed to grape flavor and it was quite different to the actual cigarette flavor, because the tobacco vape doesn't taste like a cigarette at all [...] when I started using the grape flavor [...] my mind can separate the two, vaping/smoking, so it's sort of why I think it helped me move away from that*" (FG1M3).

Concerning awareness of nicotine presence in e-liquids and related relevance, five participants were aware of it (4 dual users and 1 ENDS user) and four were not (2 hookah users, 1 ENDS user, and 1 dual user). Notably, one hookah user was not aware of nicotine presence in tobacco used in hookahs: "*Because, when I used to smoke, that was like free of nicotine, just the flavor thing so [...] that was like ok, not much harm that I'm doing.*" Moreover, when asked about the importance of nicotine presence in e-liquids, most of the participants (7) found nicotine critical, for example, "*I mean for the most part doesn't matter the flavor, there is no vape purpose if there is not nicotine, [...]. There's not really much point doing it, without the nicotine*" (FG1M3). Nevertheless, for some participants nicotine was a matter of concern, for example, "*I usually try to get non-nicotine. I'm just trying to not get addicted to nicotine*" (FG2M1). In addition, for the second hookah, user nicotine content was not as important as it was flavor.

The levels of nicotine more frequently used by participants varied between low (0–3 mg/ml) to very high (salts) >18 mg/ml. One dual user compared his nicotine addiction to caffeine addiction: "*I would most often buy the lowest, which is 3 mg/ml, and that's down to like I am addicted to nicotine but in the same way that someone is addicted to caffeine. Like you would not go in the morning without a cup of coffee just because you do not want to and so I choose the nicotine option*" (FG4M1). Another dual user associated levels of nicotine used to circumstance: "*I usually use 6 mg/ml, I also use 50 mg or 30 mg [...], because [I] jump onto the top occasionally if I'm just stressed out, but because I do that I don't know the exact amount when I do that*" (FG1M3). In addition, two dual users were taken by surprise when they learned about different levels of nicotine in e-liquids: "*I never considered that, because I never thought that there would be different levels of nicotine, or that you can get it free of nicotine. I picked fruity flavors because I like them, but if I knew, I'd prefer the ones with lower nicotine*" (FG3F1); "*Even the mint ones will have nicotine on it? oh*" (FG1M1). In addition, two participants indicated not having a vaping device, adducing that when needed they could just use their friend's, for example, "*If I wanted to use, I could use somebody else's*" (FG2M1).

When asked about places for vaping, more than actual locations, answers related to a situation: hanging out with friends (7 participants), for example, "*If you are doing it alone, that's sad*" (FG3M2). Associated locations were at home (2), in a bar (2) outside (2), shisha bar (2), anywhere (2), and in the car (1). Some relevant statements included: "*In the car mostly. Because then you don't have to take time out of your day. [...]. It's quite fun to take to parties and stuff, stops you from smoking cigarettes at a party. If I'm like out drinking and smoking cigarettes I can [go] through like 5 or 6 [cigarettes] and it's quite expensive*" (FG4M1). "*If I'm just walking down the street then I would have had a smoke or if I'm waiting somewhere, vaping is [...] quick, you just sort of do it, wherever. If you got a cigarette, it's a time constraint as well because you're like burn it, it takes a couple of minutes, the vape is two seconds*" (FG1M3). Additionally, some frustrations about current bar smoking/vaping rules and settings were stated: "*Lots of bars I don't quite like because if somebody is trying to vape exclusively and [don't want] to come back to the cigarette, you are sort of forced into the cigarette area [...]*" (FG1M2). Interestedly, some participants (5) found sharing devices, a commonly accepted practice, for example, "*I mean sometimes, if I'm at a party, somehow it gets around [...] I really don't have a problem with that as long as it returns to me, no one breaks it*" (FG1M3).

3.5 Triggers: situations or feelings that triggered cravings for vaping

Regarding visual stimuli acting as a vaping trigger (e.g., seeing others vaping), four dual users answered that it does not. Conversely, seeing others smoking tobacco cigarettes can be a trigger for smoking, for example, "*Vaping does not really trigger me, smoking does trigger me for smoking*" (FG1M2). Two participants found some association, for example, "*... If I see other people vape, I feel more inclined to do it*" (FG2M1); "*I think that depends on the situation and where I am. The other day [in] a bar there were people vaping, I felt the temptation of vaping, but when I'm walking to the university and I see other people vaping I do not feel the need, because I'm coming here to study so my focus is on the studies I don't feel tempted then*" (FG3F1). Moreover, one dual user indicated that the ENDS "artificial" look causes him to have a mental block "*... For me, it's so robotic, the vape, it doesn't have the organic, I mean the cigarettes are still a plant, still lights, but vape, just feel like you are taking a machine into your body, like in a hospital kind of thing, you're check in for the machine. Maybe for me, that's part of the mental block: sure, you got the nicotine hit, but it looks too artificial. I feel, no men no*" (FG1M1). Concerning the smell of e-liquids acting as cravings triggers, only three participants (1 dual user, 1 hookah user, and 1 ENDS user) were positive, for example, "*I prefer the smell of fruit, so, when I smell cigarettes, I don't feel tempted, but with fruity vapes, I do feel the temptation to try again*" (FG3F1). In addition, vaping advertising or vaping shops did not trigger vaping cravings.

To the question of stressful situations acting as vaping triggers, three participants found some association to unspecified stressful situations, for example, "*If things are not great, I probably will be vaping a lot more. It's a coping response. Again, and then it becomes this point there's bigger things to worry about yeah, right?*" (FG1M2). Moreover, two participants may use either, under highly stressful situations, for example, "*It kind of depends on how I feel like at the time, but also like the severity of it. So, if I just had like a really traumatic event I probably just go straight and have a cigarette but like I mean, the same effect from vaping, but cigarettes are just quicker and stronger*" (FG4M1). Two participants also found studying a stress-related vaping trigger. The remaining participants did not find any relation.

When exploring deeper, views regarding the role of social contexts as vaping triggers, four participants' (3 dual users and 1 ENDS user) answers were affirmative, for example, "*It's like the worst, being the [odd] one out [...] everyone is smoking and you are not smoking. For sure if anyone is passing around a machine, I want a piece of the machine*" (FG1M1). On the other hand, one dual user who previously lived overseas noted that, since he moved to NZ, smoking and vaping has changed from a very socially driven practice to a very lonely experience: "*now it has become like the completely solitary thing it used to be a very special thing, very social thing ... but that doesn't happen that often [now]*" (FG1M2). The fact that vaping can be seen as a solitary practice was also shared by another dual user. In addition, one dual user found that social situations might not necessarily represent a trigger factor or a reason to vape: "*Probably [socializing] doesn't really make a difference. So, I just got a vape when I feel like it and sometimes, I might be around a crowd of friends, that none of them vape or smoke, so to that event I wouldn't bring my vape, but other times yeah, [I will] be going out maybe [with] people that I'm going with vape or smokes, and so I bring my vape along*" (FG4M1). For the hookah users, rather being than a trigger, socializing was a situation in which, in order to hang out, vaping was compulsory: "*being in a party, I used to do it. If I didn't do it, it would be like turned down from the group [...] So we have to participate, even if you have only one drag, you have to, it's the kind of thing*" (FG3M2).

3.6 Reactions and views associated with vaping: Moods, benefits, harms to health, smoking vs. vaping, quitting smoking, participants' plans to quit vaping

Seven participants indicated feeling relaxed, as the mood most associated with vaping, followed by: happy (4 participants), focused (2), and stimulated (1). Some participants indicated more than one mood associated with vaping, for example, "*All of the time it's relaxing. Some of the time it can cheer you up, if you are just a bit moody that day or whatever, go for really nice vape [and] you're happier because of it*" (FG4M1). The same participant voiced some concern: "*In terms of vaping you don't seem to have that finish point [as] with a cigarette [...], with vaping it's not. [Instead it's] 'give me another hit, give me another hit', kind of thing. That is a big negative of vaping for me because I can see myself just sitting [vaping]*" (FG1M1). Nevertheless, in relation to the benefits found with vaping, several reasons stand out: making friends, a feeling of belonging, peace, fun, it helps work better, psychological control, and it does not interfere with daily activities, such as working out as much as cigarettes can do.

The perceptions associated with harm to health from vaping vs. harm caused by smoking tobacco cigarettes were as follows: six participants found vaping less harmful than smoking cigarettes, and for two others more data/research is needed to determine vaping's long-term health risk. One believed that vaping is as harmful as smoking tobacco cigarettes and for other, vaping represented a risk due to the e-liquid intake: "*For me, that would be a big risk of vaping, you seem to be a seat in a trap, you seat there a lot more, take a lot more on*" (FG1M1). In addition, when asked about their opinion on whether using both (ENDS and tobacco cigarettes) was healthier than only smoking tobacco cigarettes, four dual users answer yes, and one (dual user) said that using both, although it may help regulating and cutting down smoking and use of tobacco cigarettes, may have a nicotine addictive effect. One hookah user indicated that using both is less healthy than smoking only, and two more participants considered the opposite.

Dual users were asked about how ENDS helped them to quit smoking tobacco cigarettes. For this, two participants re-stated their relapses. In one case, the participant had recently managed to quit smoking for 3 months before relapsing. Another had managed to exclusively vape for several months, after earlier relapses. A third one acknowledged a failure in this regard: "*Nah, failed [I] started 10 years ago, it didn't work. Now I thought about trying again, [but] it hasn't work[ed].*" For some others, quitting smoking by using ENDS can only happen with discipline: "*It alleviates the cravings pretty quick. Like, you only need to do like one puff really, to stop smoking a cigarette, so it's quite effective in that regard. It feels like, if you were trying to cut out the smoking, then you need to be quite disciplined with the vaping because it's pretty easy to pick up the vape and vape more than you should.*" Moreover, when asked about how satisfying vaping was, six participants felt satisfied, from which two (dual users) commented: "*To save a lot of money, exactly. Yeah, like I said before, I love it. I feel a little bit less tired. Like the stomach upset wise, my throat feels a little bit better than when I was smoking [only] and again comes down to right now I just don't care enough, I think you really need to care about your health at some point if you want to quit smoking*" (FG1M2). "*For me, it's been a financial benefit [...] I guess it has brought a social benefit in the sense that I don't feel the need to [smoke]. So, [it's] mainly financially better for me, and obviously, some health benefit, because there was a period when I was heavily smoking for a while but I just can't taste anything...*" (FG1M3). Despite being positive, another dual user voiced concerns: "*I think that it's a good alternative, and especially as there's more research into it. I think that the ban on the nice flavors is probably a good idea because I don't like the idea, myself included, that people just vape for fun, because it's just a good way to get really addicted to nicotine [...], so if you are using it to cut out the cigarettes, I think it's a good alternative.*" On the contrary, one person did not find it satisfactory: "*I don't know, it just feels like, a waste of money you don't get much for it [...]. I don't enjoy it as much ...*" (FG2M1).

In regards to recommending vaping as a way to quit smoking tobacco cigarettes, mixed opinions were given: for three participants it was an option, for example, "*I think it's a good alternative because it gets you a lot more control over exactly how much nicotine you get.*" Three other participants had doubts, for example, "*I do n't know about it because I've got so many mates, including myself, who tried to quit that way they bought it and they haven't. So, for me to recommend that to someone seems a bit disingenuous.*" Moreover, one participant would recommend it as a way to help reduce the tobacco cigarettes intake. Another one recommended it with warnings: "*I feel like if somebody is at the point where they start really caring, then I'll tell you to use a vape to try to quit. For me it [has been] such a rollercoaster [...] you need to know a lot of things before you start this and if you pick wrong on the nicotine level, you might hit your tolerance like crazy it's very tempting to always do it [...] like I've gone to hell and back with my tolerance based on vaping*" (FG1M2).

The final question asked, was related to plans to quit vaping, to which only one participant considered quitting a possibility: "*Yeah, probably. I don't do it much at the moment [...]. Well, likely to do it [...] my friends are stopping doing it [...] I'll see*" (FG2M1). Four participants were not considering quitting in the foreseeable future, for different reasons, such as occasional use (1 hookah user) and intermittent use (1 dual user), do not consider nicotine addiction as a bad thing (1 dual user): "*I mean, probably not [quitting], just because I don't really see having a nicotine addiction as a bad thing [...]. I enjoy it, and I think probably right now it brings me more benefits to my life than the negatives [...], the whole reason for vaping in the first place is for the nicotine*" (FG1M3). The final related statement was: "*Now, like I said that's one of the things I would really need to [quit], and I know that, but that doesn't mean that [it] can change for the foreseeable future I don't think so. When I get off the nicotine, I'm not functional at all, and that's the big issue right now*" (FG1M2).

After finishing covering all focus groups' topics, the recording systems were turned off and all participants were thanked for their participation and were asked any further questions about the project and the focus groups discussions.

4. Discussion

Analyzing the participants' demographics, the cultural and ethnic diversity of the group was evident. Their diverse backgrounds allowed us to have a glimpse into different geographical and cultural contexts surrounding ENDS use. Cultural and geographical contexts should be considered when working toward the development of more targeted and personalized VRT and telehealth services, since they may influence the subject's level of immersion and sense of presence during a VR intervention and, therefore, their physiological and psychological responses [17]. While the resulting information from the number of participants interviewed does not provide a comprehensive representation of the vaping community in NZ, it shows some of the varied factors influencing vaping in our universities. A limited number of participants has not been an impediment to carry out similar qualitative studies in the past [18]. In our study, despite a comprehensive recruitment campaign, only a small turnout of candidates was obtained. Nevertheless, the information acquired not only has provided valuable insights from the participants' perspectives but also has contributed toward gaining a better understanding of how students from diverse backgrounds adapt their vaping habits for NZ university contexts. Statements gathered in these focus group discussions will contribute toward VRS development that resembles more accurately situations and environments related to vaping among young people.

The financial benefit when compared to smoking tobacco cigarettes was the main reason why the participants started vaping. It is remarkable how the lower prices of vaping products influenced the participants' transition toward a more affordable source of nicotine. While higher taxes on tobacco products may be associated with a decline in tobacco smoking, conversely, it may have also influenced the increase in ENDS use [19]. In this regard, before making any assumptions, it is important to consider that, although ENDS have been promoted as a less harmful option than conventional tobacco, there are increasing concerns regarding their long-term health risks, which are already a matter of public health debate [20]. Advance long-term studies are needed to come to definitive conclusions [21]. Furthermore, our findings about the reasons why the participants continued using ENDS were associated mainly with two factors: nicotine and flavor. Together with the perception that ENDS are less harmful to health, these have been identified previously as some of the main reasons why vaping are so popular among teens and young adults [22, 23].

While vaping has become a viable nicotine alternative to many, for some of our dual users, ENDS did not satisfy completely their needs, and stopping smoking tobacco cigarettes was not seen as an option in the foreseeable future. Compared to tobacco cigarettes, ENDS deliver lower levels of plasma nicotine, which can produce an unsatisfied feeling in dual users, inducing them to increase their nicotine intake, either by smoking, vaping, or using more of both [24]. Thus, some dual users may face not only nicotine dependency issues but also potential health problems, such as respiratory and heart conditions [24]. Noticeably, quitting smoking was not found to be one of the main reasons to start vaping, similar to other studies [25, 26], where health, curiosity, or financial reasons had a more relevant role in making the decision. In addition, some dual users in our study indicated having a recurrent pattern of intermittent phases between tobacco cigarettes and vaping and/or using both during the same period. In a recent study [23], similar transitions from single to dual or from dual to single-use were described in one out of three study participants, who were all adolescents (13–18 years old). In our study, the majority of participants were young adults and the pattern described here was spontaneously stated by them rather than being a pre-established assessment.

In regards to e-liquids of choice, as previously established among youth, young adults, and adult vapers [5, 27], flavored products were the most popular ones, among our study's participants. Moreover, in relation to flavors, fruit e-liquids were preferred, followed by menthol, as has been reported previously [28]. Similar to the findings of a recent survey carried out in North America [29], tobacco flavor was not popular, but rather was considered unpleasant. As indicated, flavored e-liquids have become topics of research and discussion since they are determinant factors for vaping initiation and may act as a gateway to smoking cigarettes and nicotine dependency [30–32]. Regardless of the source, nicotine dependency has been associated with disturbances of cognitive development in teens and young adults [33]. In addition, recent studies have reported the presence of toxic substances in vape aerosols [34] and the findings of traces of some chemicals in menthol mint and fruit-flavored e-liquids that increase the risk of cancer [22]. Nevertheless, in some cases, flavored e-liquids have been reported to help some users to cut down on tobacco smoking [35], as was reported by one of our participants. In this regard, the use of flavored e-liquids has been suggested for use in self-help for smoking cessation, alongside other intervention types, such as educational videogames [36, 37], which may be further developed toward targeted VR and telehealth.

In this study, nicotine (the presence and level of) was a determining factor for vaping among some participants (mainly dual users). Notably, other participants manifested a lack of awareness about nicotine information in the e-liquid that they have used. Moreover, in some cases, the participants stated a lack of knowledge on whether or not the products they tried contained nicotine. Neither did they know about the nicotine levels of their preferred products, similar to previous findings [38]. Although consumer awareness is required in many countries, limitations in users' knowledge about vaping products may be associated with the lack of proper warning labels for e-liquids and even mislabeling in some cases [38]. This should be a matter of concern, particularly since the population at higher risk to start using ENDS are teens and young adults. Not only should correct labeling be mandatory but also educational tools for information and guidance should be available for all current and potential users. In this regard, the NZ government is making an effort to regulate all vaping and smokeless tobacco through the Smokefree Environments and Regulated Products Act, 1990 [11]. VRT and telehealth can be used as platforms for prevention and education for all potential health risks associated with vaping.

Hanging out with friends was a situation highly linked to vaping for our focus group participants. Notably for the hookah users interviewed, when hanging out with friends back in their country of origin, at times when vaping took place, this was considered a must-do activity among them. Thus, similar to the findings of previous studies [14, 39], it appears that among our participants, vaping is predominantly a social practice and is increasingly more socially accepted. Moreover, for some participants, it may be part of their socio-cultural practices. In some cases, as a social practice, sharing ENDS devices among friends was considered acceptable, and because of this, some participants did not consider it necessary to acquire their own devices, as long as sharing was an option. Conversely, in a study developed with students of the

University of Edinburgh, sharing ENDS was considered socially unacceptable [40], depending on temporal and geographical contexts. In addition, it was notable how vaping, unlike smoking cigarettes, was perceived as a more flexible practice that conveniently can be integrated into different situations or places, such as being in a bar, at home, studying, walking, or driving, either within social or individual contexts. Similar findings were reported by Keane et al. [14]. Nevertheless, the culture shock experienced by some of our international students seemed to have influenced their vaping behavior and attitudes toward it, since either the social context or the physical settings experienced in NZ do not match what they were familiar with, in their country of origin. This reinforces the idea that ENDS contexts and characteristics vary according to culture and geographical location.

In relation to vaping triggers, unlike previous reports [41], in our study, neither passive exposure to vaping nor vaping advertisement appeared to trigger a desire for vaping or smoking. This applies mainly to dual users, who also indicated that, when seeing others smoking tobacco cigarettes, this may trigger their desire for smoking, which sometimes, maybe mitigated with vaping [42]. In terms of olfactory triggers, only fruit e-liquids were found to have some effect. With respect to the role of stressful situations as vaping craving triggers, it seems that regardless of the nature of it, for some of our participants, vaping may be used as a coping mechanism for stress. Similar findings were observed by tobacco cigarette users, which may be associated with nicotine [43]. Moreover, some of our participants related vaping to feeling relaxed, happier, focused, stimulated, and responses that have been linked previously to the effect of nicotine [44]. In addition, a highlighted concern raised by some participants was related to a perception of losing control over vape intake and "endless" vaping. Similar remarks have been observed in for dual users and young adults [40]. This may be associated to previous user's sense of having control over their own smoking, given by the knowledge of time taken to smoke a conventional tobacco cigarette. Nevertheless, uninhibited vaping may induce to higher consumption of nicotine, which given the ever-growing popularity of vaping, may contribute to an overall increase in nicotine dependency, therefore, higher health risks.

In general, our participants perceived vaping as a less harmful practice than smoking conventional cigarettes. Even though the long-term health effects of vaping are under investigation, the same impression seems to be shared by many [36, 45, 46]. The majority of participants considered the use of both ENDS and smoking conventional cigarettes healthier than to smoke tobacco cigarettes only. Although there is insufficient scientific evidence to support this statement, the perception may be associated with the idea that cigarette consumption may be reduced, despite its continued use of it [46, 47]. It is important to remember that vaping and its potential harmful effects depend on many factors, such as frequency of use, the quantity of nicotine consumed, flavors of preference, and type of devices used, together with socioeconomic and associated demographic factors. In particular vaping practice has been associated with youth in socioeconomic disadvantage, who have never smoked [46], which may serve as a gateway to nicotine dependency and consequently, associated health issues. An integrated analysis of contexts and factors influencing vaping is needed to advance effective future interventions and treatments for vaping disorders. As for the lack of success in trying to quit smoking by vaping, it appears to be a common situation among college students and adults [36, 48], who either fail, relapse, or become dual users. It appears that for some participants of our study, relapsing may be a common situation and for others, quitting smoking seems to be a challenge only achievable by being extremely disciplined. As the effectiveness of using vaping to quit smoking appears to be debatable [46], vaping may be of better use as a tool to help reduce smoking. Some attributes associated with vaping, such as being more socially accepted, the variety of e-liquids flavors as well as different levels of nicotine concentration, may be of help in the effort to reduce smoking [39], nevertheless, the potential effect caused by these attributes should be carefully considered.

In general, our participants seemed to be satisfied with vaping. This feeling was primarily linked to its financial benefit compared to smoking, followed by health and social acceptance. As mentioned by some of our participants, due to high taxation on cigarettes it is possible that, in NZ, conventional cigarette smokers are switching to vaping, a situation that may have been further enhanced by health marketing campaigns [13]. How this may have affected the use of vaping by non-smokers and possibly influenced the increase in nicotine dependency is yet to be understood and is critical to be quantified. The questions about recommending vaping as a way to quit smoking conventional cigarettes, varied opinions were obtained in our focus groups. Our participants' views agree with other studies' report, in which vapers did not recommend it due to their own or their friends' failed attempts [40], or even their own difficulties and struggles with self-controlling nicotine intake. In addition, regarding plans to quit vaping, there was not a clear position about it. Whether it is because of the benefits seen by using it (when compared to smoking conventional cigarettes), nicotine dependency, or their occasional use, quitting vaping does not appear to be considered a priority in the foreseeable future for most of our participants.

As observed in this study, vaping is a dynamic practice. The discussions that took place throughout our focus group sessions, provided important information that has helped us to identify some key social, cultural, and economic components in the vaping contexts of a diverse group of young adults. This material will contribute to the development of a more realistic and immersive VRS. The current technological advances achieved in the development of online VRS can enable better integration with telehealth for the future delivery of interventions and treatments as well as prevention and education campaigns for vaping-related disorders. This would build on recent developments using VRT in telemental health services, in areas, such as social anxiety, obsessive-compulsive and substance use disorders [49], and smoking interventions [50]. As yet, the knowledge of vaping-related disorders is limited and still a work in progress. Nevertheless, the use of VRT for cue exposure treatments could represent an alternative to help patients suffering from nicotine dependence caused by vaping. Moreover, in order to help achieve better results, previous studies developed in smoking cue exposure therapy using VRT have recommended, including mechanisms that help patients to improve their coping skills [7, 51]. In addition, studies indicate a potential need to modulate negative effects and stress during cue exposure [7]. These recommendations are worth being considered and testing in future vaping treatments using VRT.

5. Limitations

The limitations of the study were primarily related to the number of vapers interviewed in the focus groups and how representative the sample could be in relation to different types of vapers, given demographic factors and geographic location. Thus, we acknowledge that our findings are limited to the views, background, behavior, and environments surrounding a sample of local and international university students in

NZ. Nevertheless, despite how dynamic and rapidly growing vaping is, in our study, we found similarities with some perceptions and behaviors described in previous studies carried out worldwide [5, 14, 22, 23, 27, 38, 39], which help to support our findings and will contribute toward vaping-related VRS development.

6. Conclusion

In this study, the accessible price of vaping products was a key reason for starting and continuing vaping. In most cases, vaping was associated with nicotine dependency by the participants, particularly for dual users. In our sample, flavored e-liquids were popular, especially fruit and menthol, but not tobacco flavor. Flavored e-liquids may be seen to help with the transition from smoking conventional tobacco into vaping, but they are also a concern for potential nicotine dependency. Furthermore, in this group, vaping appears to be mostly seen as a social practice, linked to hanging out with friends, regardless of the location (party, bar, house, car, etc.). On the other hand, for some international students, their current settings for vaping are dissimilar to what they were used to in their countries of origin, which, in some cases, has led to a change in vaping behaviors from a social context into a solitary practice.

In our study, passive exposure to vaping or vaping advertisements appears not to be a trigger for vaping or smoking but for dual users, seeing others smoking conventional cigarettes does trigger their desire for smoking conventional cigarettes, which may not always be mitigated by vaping. When compared to smoking, vaping is perceived as more socially accepted, healthier, more beneficial, and in general satisfying. Moreover, while vaping was not perceived as a way to quit smoking, it may be of help to reduce smoking conventional cigarettes, but concerns remained regarding a tendency toward loss of control of nicotine intake that can occur when vaping, which may induce nicotine dependence. Nevertheless, quitting vaping does not seem to be a concern or priority among our participants, and this may lead to continued or even increased nicotine dependency as well as increasing the risk of health disorders associated with vaping. Further studies are needed to clarify and test these matters.

Vaping is an ever-changing global practice with rapid technological and social growth, which may be taking nicotine dependency to a new level, reaching all socio-cultural contexts and age groups. The socio-cultural and economic background of the target population should become a key component to be considered when developing new technological tools toward enabling more inclusive and personalized online VRT and telehealth services for prevention, intervention, and treatment of vaping and its potential associated disorders. The dynamic and multifactorial character of vaping together with its potential associated health risks makes it a key challenge for future VRT and telehealth developments. Furthermore, as adolescents and young adults are at higher risk, the use of online VRT for telehealth represents an attractive and accessible technological platform that can be used to engage this age group to be better informed about vaping. Further technological advancements should facilitate interactive access to online environments developed under more realistic and contextualized settings, in which prevention, control, and treatment focused telehealth programs can tackle commonly associated issues, such as nicotine dependence, ENDS misuse, health harms linked to e-liquids flavors and chemical components. Thus, further developments in online VRS are needed to enhance and facilitate telehealth services in the growing field of vaping-related disorders.

Acknowledgements

We thank the Health Research Council of New Zealand (HRC), for the explorer grant number 17/738 that funded this project.

We would like to thank Nawan Karki who contributed with technical support to carry out the focus group sessions by looking after the video and audio settings. We are grateful to M.D. Wilson for proofreading the manuscript.

Conflict of interest

The authors declare no conflict of interest.

Author details

Maria Cecilia Vega-Corredor[1*], Simon Hoermann[2,3], Alison Watkins[1] and Melanie Tomintz[1]

1 Geospatial Research Institute, University of Canterbury, Christchurch, New Zealand

2 School of Product Design, University of Canterbury, Christchurch, New Zealand

3 HIT Lab NZ, University of Canterbury, Christchurch, New Zealand

*Address all correspondence to: maria.vegacorredor@canterbury.ac.nz

References

[1] Adkison SE, O'Connor RJ, Bansal-Travers M, Hyland A, Borland R, Yong H, et al. Electronic nicotine delivery systems. American Journal of Preventive Medicine. 2013;**44**(3):207-215. DOI: 10.1016/j.amepre.2012.10.018

[2] Olonoff M, Niaura R, Hitsman B. Electronic cigarettes are not cigarettes, and why that matters. Nicotine & Tobacco Research. 2019;**21**(10):1441-1444. DOI: 10.1093/ntr/nty205

[3] Chadi N, Hadland SE, Harris SK. Understanding the implications of the vaping epidemic among adolescents and young adults: A call for action. Substance Abuse. 2019;**40**(1):7-10

[4] Oriakhi M. Vaping: An emerging health hazard. Cureus. 2020;**12**:3. DOI: 10.7759/cureus.7421

[5] Zare S, Nemati M, Zheng Y. A systematic review of consumer preference for e-cigarette attributes: Flavor, nicotine strength, and type. PLoS One. 2018;**133**:e0194145. DOI: 10.1371/journal.pone.0194145

[6] Kisker J, Gruber T, Schöne B. Behavioral realism and lifelike psychophysiological responses in virtual reality by the example of a height exposure. Psychological Research Psychologische Forschung. 2019;**85**(1):68-81. DOI: 10.1007/s00426-019-01244-9

[7] Pericot-Valverde I, Secades-Villa R, Gutiérrez-Maldonado J. A randomized clinical trial of cue exposure treatment through virtual reality for smoking cessation. Journal of Substance Abuse Treatment. 2019;**96**:26-32. DOI: 10.1016/j.jsat.2018.10.003

[8] Kamińska D, Sapiński T, Wiak S, Tikk T, Haamer R, Avots E, et al. Virtual reality and its Alications in education: Survey. Information (Basel). 2019;**10**(10):318. DOI: 10.3390/info10100318

[9] Tamplin J, Loveridge B, Clarke K, Li Y, Berlowitz D. Development and feasibility testing of an online virtual reality platform for delivering therapeutic group singing interventions for people living with spinal cord injury. Journal of Telemedicine and Telecare. 2020;**26**(6):365-375. DOI: 10.1177/1357633X19828463

[10] Gurram N. Electronic cigarette online marketing by New Zealand vendors. New Zealand Medical Journal. 2019;**132**(1506):20-33

[11] Ministry of Health, New Zealand. Regulation of vaping and smokeless tobacco products [internet]. 2022. Available from: https://www.health.govt.nz/our-work/regulation-health-and-disability-system/regulation-vaping-and-smokeless-tobacco-products. [Accessed: April 07, 2022]

[12] Ministry of Health, New Zealand. Daily youth smoking rates at all time low in Aotearoa Media release 28 February 2022 [Internet]. 2022. Available from: https://www.health.govt.nz/news-media/media-releases/daily-youth-smoking-rates-all-time-low-aotearoa. [Accessed: April 07, 2022]

[13] Health Promotion Agency NZ. Vaping facts: Vape to Quit campaign coming [Internet]. 2021. Available from: https://newsletter.hpa.org.nz/campaigns/reports/viewCampaignaspx?d=r&c=BAE1E0C2C9F2C8BA&ID=FF7430872482511B2540EF23F30FEDED&temp=False&tx=0&source=Report [Accessed: April 07, 2022]

[14] Keane H, Weier M, Fraser D, Gartner C. 'Anytime, anywhere': Vaping as social practice. Critical Public Health. 2017;**27**(4):465-476. DOI: 10.1080/09581596.2016.1250867

[15] Corbin JM, Strauss AL. Basics of Qualitative Research: Techniques and Procedures for Developing Grounded Theory. 4th ed. Thousand Oaks: SAGE; 2015. p. 456

[16] Lopez D, Whitehead D. Sampling data and data collection in qualitative research. In: Schneider Z, Whitehead D, Lobiondo-Wood G, Haber J, editors. Nursing and Midwifery Research Methods and Appraisal for Evidence Practice. 4th ed. Sydney: Elsevier; 2013. pp. 123-140

[17] Gorini A, Mosso JL, Mosso D, Pineda E, Ruíz NL, Ramíez M, et al. Emotional response to virtual reality exposure across different cultures: The role of the attribution process. Cyberpsychology & Behaviour. 2009;**2**(6):699-705. DOI: 10.1089/cpb.2009.0192

[18] Barbeau AM, Burda J, Siegel M. Perceived efficacy of e-cigarettes versus nicotine replacement therapy among successful e-cigarette users: A qualitative approach. Addiction Science & Clinical Practice. 2013;**8**(1):5-5. DOI: 10.1186/1940-0640-8-5

[19] Pesko MF, Courtemanche CJ, Maclean J. The effects of traditional cigarette and e-cigarette tax rates on adult tobacco product use. Journal of Risk and Uncertainty. 2020;**60**(3):229-258. DOI: 10.1007/s11166-020-09330-9

[20] Prochaska JJ. The public health consequences of e-cigarettes: A review by the National Academies of sciences a call for more research, a need for regulatory action. Addiction. 2019;**114**(4):587-589. DOI: 10.1111/add.14478

[21] National Academies of Sciences Engineering and Medicine, Health and Medicine Division, Board on Population Health and Public Health Practice. Committee on the review of the health effects of electronic nicotine delivery systems. In: Eaton DL, Kwan LY, Stratton K, editors. Public Health Consequences of E-Cigarettes. Washington: National Academies Press; 2018. p. 774. DOI: 10.17226/24952

[22] Dinardo P, Rome ES. Vaping: The new wave of nicotine addiction. Cleveland Clinic Journal of Medicine. 2019;**861**(2):789-798. DOI: 10.3949/ccjm.86a.19118

[23] Vogel EA, Prochaska JJ, Ramo DE, Rubinstein AJ, ML. Adolescents' E-cigarette use: Increases in frequency, dependence, and nicotine exposure over 12 months. Journal of Adolescent Health. 2019;**64**(6):770-775. DOI: 10.1016/j.jadohealth.2019.02.019

[24] Wang JB, Olgin JE, Nah G, Vittinghoff E, Cataldo JK, Pletcher MJ, et al. Cigarette and e-cigarette dual use and risk of cardiopulmonary symptoms in the Health eHeart study. PLoS One. 2018;**13**(7):e0198681-e0198681. DOI: 10.1371/journal.pone.0198681

[25] Cooper M, Harrell MB, Perry CL. Comparing young adults to older adults in e-cigarette perceptions and motivations for use: Implications for health communication. Health Education Research. 2016;**31**(4):429-438. DOI: 10.1093/her/cyw030

[26] Lewek P, Woźniak B, Maludzińska P, Śmigielski J, Kardas P. Polish e-cigarettes: Users reasons to start vaping – A survey of 1142 polish vapers. Family Medicine & Primary Care Review. 2018;**20**(3):232-235. DOI: 10.5114/FMPCR.2018.78257

[27] Harrel MC, Bradley MA. Data Collection Methods: Semi-Structured

Interviews and Focus Groups. Santa Monica: RAND; 2009. p. 140

[28] Groom AL, Vu TT, Kesh A, Hart JL, Walker KL, Giachello AL, et al. Correlates of youth vaping flavor preferences. Preventive Medicine Reports. 2020;**18**:01094-101094. DOI: 10.1016/j.pmedr.2020.101094

[29] Gravely S, Cummings KM, Hammond D, et al. The association of E-cigarette Flavors with satisfaction, enjoyment, and trying to quit or stay abstinent from smoking among regular adult vapers from Canada and the United States: Findings from the 2018 ITC four country smoking and vaping survey. Nicotine & Tobacco Research. 2020;**22**:1831-1841. DOI: 10.1093/ntr/ntaa095

[30] Gendall P, Hoek J. Role of flavours in vaping uptake and cessation among New Zealand smokers and non-smokers: A cross-sectional study. Tobacco Control. 2021;**30**:108-110

[31] Dai H, Hao J. Flavored electronic cigarette use and smoking among youth. Pediatrics (Evanston). 2016;**138**(6):e20162513. DOI: 10.1542/peds.2016-2513

[32] Hoffman AC, Salgado RV, Dresler C, Faller RW, Bartlett C. Flavour preferences in youth versus adults: A review. Tobacco Control. 2016;**25**:ii32-ii39

[33] Sindelar JL. Regulating vaping — Policies, possibilities, and perils. The New England Journal of Medicine. 2020;**382**:e54-e54. DOI: 10.1056/NEJMp1917065

[34] Rawlinson C, Martin S, Frosina J, Wright C. Chemical characterisation of aerosols emitted by electronic cigarettes using thermal desorption–gas chromatography–time of flight mass spectrometry. Journal of Chromatography A. 2017;**1497**:144-154. DOI: 10.1016/j.chroma.2017.02.050

[35] McRobbie H, Bullen C, Hartmann-Boyce J, Hajek P. Electronic cigarettes for smoking cessation and reduction. Cochrane Database of Systematic Reviews. 2014;**12**:CD010216

[36] Camenga DR, Fiellin LE, Pendergrass T, Miller E, Pentz MA, Hieftje K. Adolescents' perceptions of flavored tobacco products, including E-cigarettes: A qualitative study to inform FDA tobacco education efforts through videogames. Addictive Behaviors. 2018;**82**:189-194. DOI: 10.1016/j.addbeh.2018.03.021

[37] Meltzer LR, Simmons VN, Piñeiro B, et al. Development of a self-help smoking cessation intervention for dual users of tobacco cigarettes and E-cigarettes. International Journal of Environmental Research and Public Health. 2021;**18**(5):2328. DOI: 10.3390/ijerph18052328

[38] Sontag JM, Wackowski OA, Hammond D. Baseline assessment of noticing e-cigarette health warnings among youth and young adults in the United States, Canada and England, and associations with harm perceptions, nicotine awareness and warning recall. Preventive Medicine Reports. 2019;**16**:100966-100966. DOI: 10.1016/j.pmedr.2019.100966

[39] Soule EK, Maloney SF, Guy MC, Eissenberg T, Fagan P. User-identified electronic cigarette behavioral strategies and device characteristics for cigarette smoking reduction. Addictive Behaviors. 2018;**79**:93-101. DOI: 10.1016/j.addbeh.2017.12.010

[40] Lucherini M, Rooke C, Amos A. They're thinking, well it's not as bad,

I probably won't get addicted to that. But it's still got the nicotine in it, so...: Maturity, control, and socializing: Negotiating identities in relation to smoking and vaping-a qualitative study of young adults in Scotland. Nicotine & Tobacco Research. 2019;**2017**(21):81-87. DOI: 10.1093/ntr/ntx245

[41] King AC, Smith LJ, Fridberg DJ, Matthews AK, McNamara PJ, Cao D. Exposure to electronic nicotine delivery systems (ENDS) visual imagery increases smoking urge and desire. Psychology of Addictive Behaviors. 2016;**30**:106-112. DOI: 10.1037/adb0000123

[42] Keijsers M, Vega-Corredor MC, Hoermann S, Tomintz M. Cue reactivity to electronic cigarettes: A systematic review. Substance Abuse: Research and Treatment. 2022;**16**:1-20. DOI: 11782218221114971

[43] Siqueira LM, Rolnitzky LM, Rickert VI. Smoking cessation in adolescents: The role of nicotine dependence, stress, and coping methods. Archives of Pediatrics & Adolescent Medicine. 2001;**155**(4):489-495. DOI: 10.1001/archpedi.155.4.489

[44] Evans DE, Drobes DJ. Nicotine self-medication of cognitive-attentional processing. Addiction Biology. 2009;**14**:32-42. DOI: 10.1111/j.1369-1600.2008.00130.x

[45] Baweja R, Curci KM, Yingst J, et al. Views of experienced electronic cigarette users. Addiction Research & Theory. 2016;**2015**(24):80-88. DOI: 10.3109/16066359.2015.1077947

[46] Green MJ, Gray L, Sweeting H, Benzeval M. Socioeconomic patterning of vaping by smoking status among UK adults and youth. BMC Public Health. 2020;**20**:183-183. DOI: 10.1186/s12889-020-8270-3

[47] Shahab L, Goniewicz ML, Blount BC, et al. Nicotine, carcinogen, and toxin exposure in long-term E-cigarette and nicotine replacement therapy users: A cross-sectional study. Annals of Internal Medicine. 2017;**166**:390-400. DOI: 10.7326/M16-1107

[48] Foulds J, Veldheer S, Berg A. Electronic cigarettes (e-cigs): Views of aficionados and clinical/public health perspectives. International Journal of Clinical Practice (Esher). 2011;**65**:1037. DOI: 10.1111/j.1742-1241.2011.02751.x

[49] Aboujaoude E, Salame W, Naim L. Telemental health: A status update. World Psychiatry. 2015;**14**:223-230. DOI: 10.1002/wps.20218

[50] Keijsers M, Vega-Corredor MC, Tomintz M, Hoermann S. Virtual reality technology use in cigarette craving and smoking interventions (I "Virtually" quit): Systematic review. Journal of Medical Internet Research. 2021;**23**(9):e24307. DOI: 10.2196/24307

[51] Budney AJ, Brown PC, Stanger C. Behavioral treatments. In: McCrady S, Epstein EE, editors. Addictions: A Comprehensive Guidebook. 2nd ed. New York: Oxford University Press; 2013. pp. 411-433

Chapter 2

Tele-electrocardiography in South-East Asia Archipelago: From a Basic Need for Healthcare Services to a Research Implementation

Idar Mappangara and Andriany Qanitha

Abstract

The fundamental principle for telemedicine implementation in the real world is to address the basic needs of healthcare services. The utilization of telemedicine naturally aimed to overcome distance, time, and financial constraints. Remote areas that are far from the cities and healthcare centers are the main regions that would mostly get benefit from the telemedicine program, for instance, in Indonesia, a country with a big archipelago area in South-East Asia. The primary healthcare center in this country is commonly available, however, the facilities and health workers are still limited. The health services are being centralized in big cities, and thus, the rural areas are far left in the context of healthcare services. Telemedicine could bring both standardized and specialized healthcare services nearer to the patients, irrespective of distance and location constraints. After receiving professional cardiology advice, implementation of telemedicine program, such as tele-electrocardiography (tele-ECG) at the primary care level, may be a financially advantageous way to identify cardiovascular disease in the general population and avoid overtreating patients. This is our first time adopting tele-ECG consultations in East Indonesia under the Makassar Telemedicine Program. This program allows us to maintain a big database of cohorts and connect its implementation to real-world clinical practices, and at the end, could guiding the health workers to improve patient's outcomes.

Keywords: tele-ECG, telemedicine, low bandwidth, click point to point, database

1. Introduction

Telemedicine, a term that appeared in the 1970s, literally means "healing at a distance" [1]. In order to improve the health of people and communities, the WHO defines telemedicine as "the delivery of healthcare services, where distance is a critical factor, by all healthcare professionals, using information and communications technologies for the exchange of valid information for the diagnosis, treatment, and prevention of disease and injuries, research and evaluation, and the continuing education of healthcare workers" [2]. As defined by the WHO, telemedicine is a system utilized to assist the healthcare functioning, especially healthcare services, education, research, and even training. The need for telemedicine is basically due to obstacles in optimizing the function of healthcare, particularly in poor-resource populations; either due to the large costs, long-distance barriers, limited human resources, the need for immediate or 24-hour services, as well as the nature of wide-spread coverage area of telemedicine [3].

The fundamental rule for managing a telemedicine program in a low- and middle-income country (LMIC) like Indonesia is whether the system can address the unmet needs for primary care services, how to deal with budgetary issues, how to empower the locals to use telemedicine, and most importantly, how to maintain and sustain the utilization for a long period of time [3]. This is often seen to be a problem or miscommunication between telemedicine-service providers who generally rely on the sophistication and completeness of the equipment, while the users on the other hand, simply ask for user-friendly devices. Unsurprisingly, the mismatch between providers' capability, supporting infrastructure, and user needs, not rarely ends up with suboptimal function, and even worse, telemedicine is not working at all [4].

2. Tele-electrocardiography in low- and middle-income countries

Electrocardiography (ECG) is one of the daily needs of healthcare services, guiding the healthcare providers such as general practitioners (GPs), nurses, and even specialists to advance their diagnosis for patients with cardiovascular complaints [5]. The use and interpretation of ECG could be challenging, especially for health workers in suburban and rural areas such as Indonesia. Moreover, the need for real-time and quick decision-making for diagnosis and treatment for patients with acute cardiovascular disease (CVD) will enforce the use of tele-ECG in limited-resource LMICs. However, the available experts to interpret the ECG, the obligation for 24/7 service and quick answers are inevitable aspects of tele-ECG, and thus, considering these important aspects is crucial to implementing tele-ECG programs in LMICs.

Tele-ECG has evolved before, during, and after this pandemic era. The tele-ECG has been instrumental in reducing the un-need patients referral and has allowed better allocation of resources through early triage of patients with acute CVD, based on their symptoms and examinations. Our previous study showed that 100% of ECG recordings were transmitted successfully and qualified for analysis; and thus, we suggest that tele-ECG can be implemented in Indonesian primary care settings with limited resources [6]. In traditional manner, when tele-ECG program was not applied, the ECG solely interpreted by the GP in the primary care center; or even worse, the ECG are not available as a basis healthcare service in several primary centers. By implementing this tele-ECG program, the consultation to the expert cardiologists may assist the GPs for immediate triage, resulting in a higher rate of early hospitalization for indicated patients, and eventually could reduce the mortality rate of acute CVD in Indonesia [6]. The flowchart of utilization and final purpose of tele-ECG is shown in **Figure 1**.

The implementation of telemedicine in LMICs may not encounter many obstacles as long as it is correlated with the needs of healthcare services, as it is fundamental to healthcare function. The first implementation of this tele-ECG program was

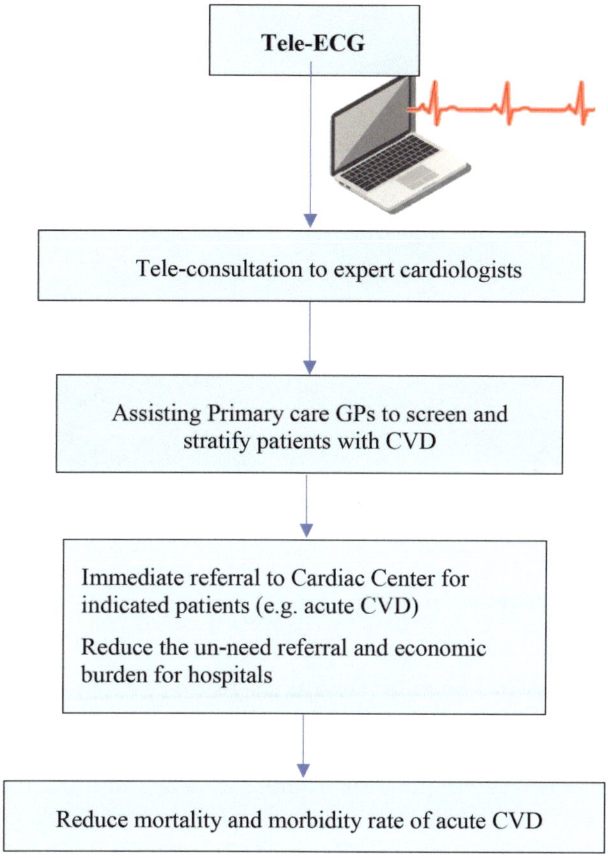

Figure 1.
The utilization and final purpose of tele-ECG program.

commenced before the Covid-19 pandemic. At that time, all patients with cardiovascular risk factors who came up to the primary care centers were screened using the tele-ECG. During this pandemic era, this tele-ECG is even more useful and practical to screen and stratify the patients with cardiac symptoms. This tele-ECG guides the GPs to determine which patients need a referral to the cardiac center, and which ones need enough observation and therapy in the primary level.

What about the research aspect? Is telemedicine program appropriate to be carried out in that direction? We agree that clinical research is important to get a big picture of the current situation of cardiology clinical practice, valuable to help analyze the real health problems and offer possible solutions to those problems. This is an interesting challenge in finding a way to implement and couple the telemedicine program with a research function.

The main principle in clinical research is that we get as much data as possible that represented the real population. The wide coverage of tele-ECG and the capability of providing big data allows the tele-ECG program as a preferable platform for conducting research. Based on our experience, conducting clinical research in LMICs is rather "exhausting." Local researchers are forced to start everything from the scratch. Unavailable standard systems for reliable databases as well as limited resources and infrastructure also contribute to the low interest and awareness of carrying out

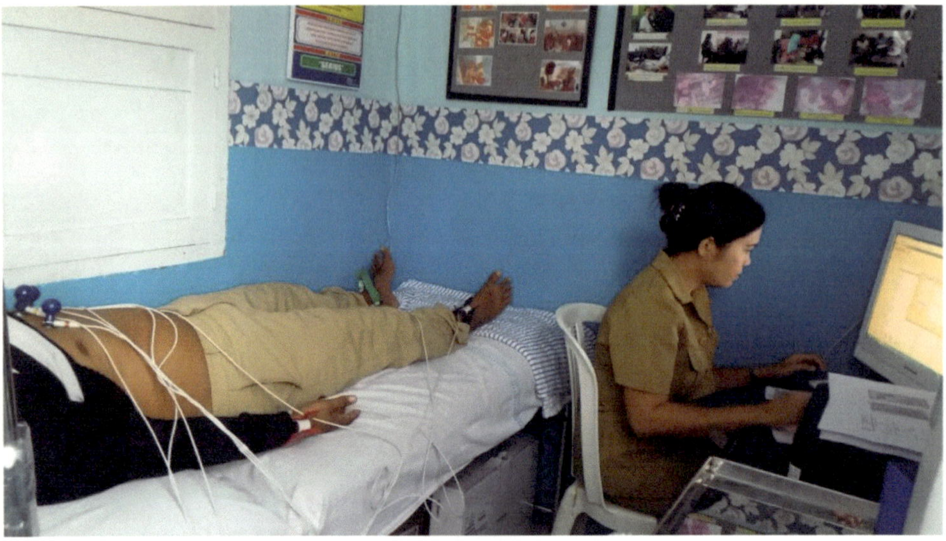

Figure 2.
Tele-ECG consultation from the primary care center.

clinical research in LMICs. **Figure 2** presents the primary care nurse performing tele-ECG consultation and contributing to a cornerstone database of tele-ECG in Indonesia.

With 17,508 islands and a population of more than 260 million, Indonesia is the most populous country in South-East Asia and the biggest archipelago in the world [7]. Java is home to more than half of Indonesia's population, with the remaining residents dispersed throughout 6000 islands [7, 8]. About 11% of the Indonesian population living in a poor socio-economic level [9]. The leading cause of mortality in this lower-middle-income country, accounting for ~37% of all fatalities, is cardiovascular disease (CVD) [9]. Despite the high burden of CVD in this country, there were only 1.5 cardiologists available per 1,000,000 people in 2016 [9] and only ~30 cardiac facilities (half of which located in Java) were available in 2013 to treat the >2.6 million prevalent cases of CAD [10, 11].

Especially in remote areas, including in some peripheral areas in Indonesia, where human resources, i.e. nurses, general practitioners, and specialist doctors are rarely available, health equipment and medical facilities are also generally inadequate and not evenly distributed. As is well known, the remote island is an area with very minimal use of technology and with all its limitations, which becomes a challenge in implementing telemedicine in archipelagic areas [12]. On this occasion, the author used the tele-ECG program as a platform to answer the challenges of implementing telemedicine in archipelagic areas, and more specifically to obtain a reliable database in terms of research function.

3. Implementing telemedicine in the archipelago region: what's the problem?

Remote islands in archipelago countries are areas that are suitable for the concept and purpose of the telemedicine program. These areas commonly live in poverty with poor health services, and urgently need assistance in solving the local health problems. To this end, telemedicine services should be utilized as routine healthcare services and function in daily practice. However, there may be challenges to run this program. In most remote areas, the healthcare officers are those with a lack knowledge and are not used to using modern technology. Mostly, medical devices in remote areas are also less modern and do not support modern application systems. In addition, in terms of infrastructure, internet signals in archipelagic areas are below average, using a low bandwidth category, and thus, a complex and sophisticated computer application in implementing telemedicine should be avoided [12].

In most LMICs, particularly in rural areas, the healthcare infrastructure is generally minimal or even unavailable, and local residents not rarely used traditional, instead of evidence-based medicine. Healthcare facilities for both diagnosis and treatment are almost blunted [13]. Based on the Speedtest Global Index, Indonesia is a country with the slowest average internet speed in Southeast Asia. As of December 2021, the average speed of mobile internet in Indonesia is only 15.44 Mbps, with the upload speed of about 9.16 Mbps, and the latency is 28 ms.

4. Telemedicine and research

The Makassar Cardiac Center launched the first telemedicine initiative in Eastern Indonesia in response to the dearth of cardiologists and the obvious demand for competence in cardiovascular treatment. With the use of this service, primary care centers can send electrocardiogram (ECG) data to Hasanuddin University Hospital. In this program, primary care GPs immediately received expertise from cardiologists when dealing with patients with CVD symptoms or risk factors. Despite the fact that Indonesia began implementing the telemedicine program in 2012, reporting on the initiative's effectiveness and results has not received as much attention.

Although telemedicine system is also developed for research functions, it is realized that research stuff is merely invaluable for the users. Primary healthcare centers and sub-health centers will certainly not be interested at all in the research objectives, especially for health workers who work on remote islands. Research appropriation is not the main issue in healthcare services in remote areas. The first and foremost is, whether the large and extensive data can be obtained through telemedicine services to improve the quality of care and clinical outcomes of patients in remote areas.

5. Telemedicine in archipelago countries: the concept of solutions

Looking at the telemedicine systems that are currently being run and developed, on average, the telemedicine system needs sophisticated technology, such as teleradiology that uses DICOM-based PACS. The telemedicine system requires modern equipment and high-speed internet with high bandwidth, which is expensive. On the other hand, to maximize telemedicine utilization, the users also should be familiar with high-tech applications. Unfortunately, these requirements are incompatible and difficult to be fulfilled in archipelagic or remote areas. Encountering these challenges and limitations, innovation and creativity are needed in designing and making an ideal and compatible telemedicine model in the archipelagic area [4, 14, 15].

The author hypothesizes that technology is flexible and can be customed to meet the local field conditions, including in extremely difficult archipelagic areas. The concept design of archipelagic telemedicine should be cheap, user-friendly and transmittable, and feasible. The design of the telemedicine system design is also should be easily utilized for the research purpose by providing reliable big data, altogether with appropriate data processing facilities, thus could be used for research and educational purposes.

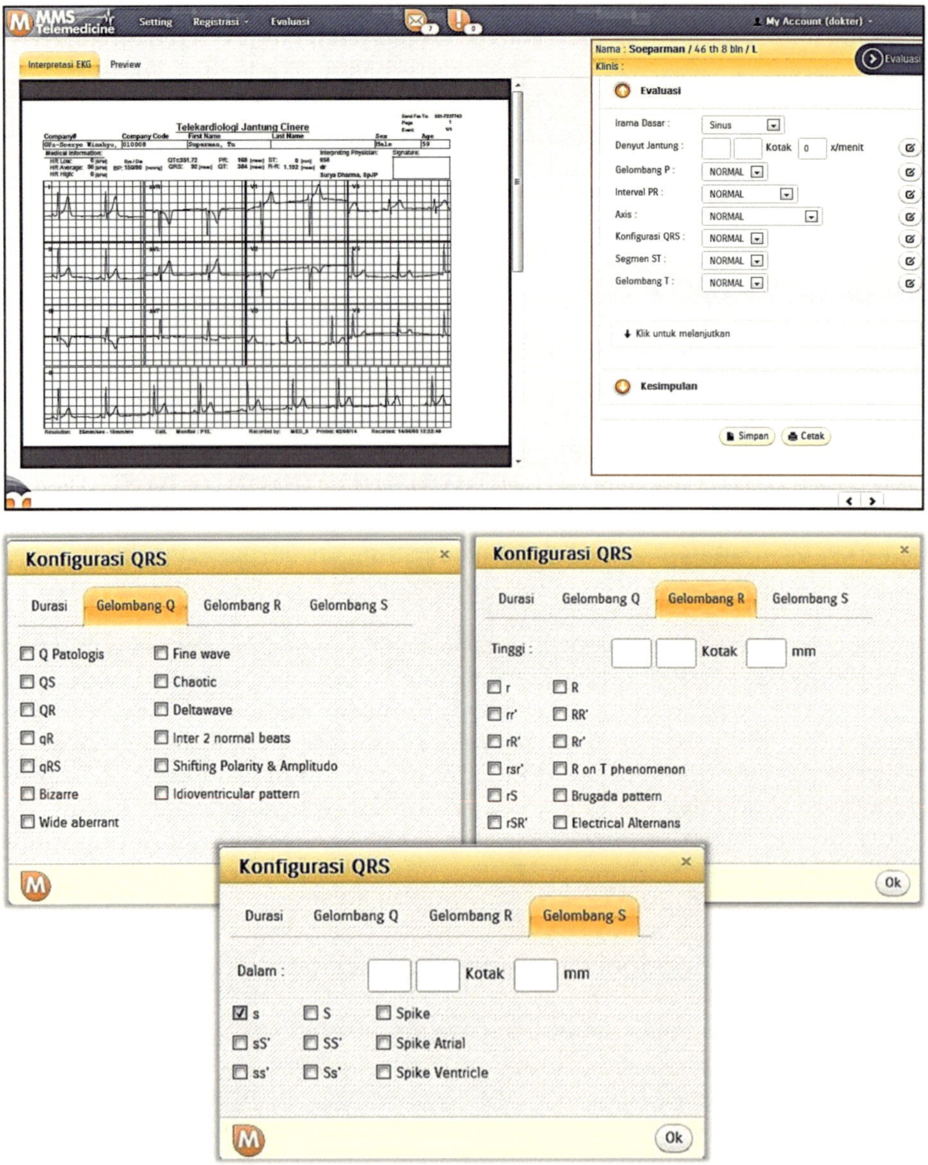

Figure 3.
Tele-ECG application used in Makassar Telemedicine Program that provides services for 46 primary care centers in Indonesia.

6. Role model of tele-ECG in Eastern Indonesia

Electrocardiography examination requires an electronic medical device called an "electrocardiogram" [5]. There are various types of tools based on the development of the system: some have DICOM-based-high-technology which is easily integrated with the current developed modern application systems, and some others are less modern and still based on non-DICOM and difficult to be integrated directly with tele-applications [4, 16–18].

In LMICs, including in Indonesia, the majority of available ECG tools is a non-DICOM-based devices. The developed tele-ECG application model will take the ECG image indirectly from the machine, and then will be stored in pdf format, as long as the ECG device has a program that could produce the output that is connectable to the computer storage, with the average size of files is less than 2 MB. This small file size is very suitable and easy to be transmitted in unstable internet speed or low-bandwidth conditions in LMICs, particularly in remote archipelagic areas. An application model with a display of the ECG image equipped with the result description on one screen will make the interpretation process by expert doctors easier.

The results and description of the ECG were made in a form of multiple choice with a point-to-point-click checklist, and thus the users will no longer need to type descriptions and conclusions of those ECG recordings. The users just need to choose the description that had been provided. The available description patterns are made by default for normal results. For example, for normal ECG results, the expert doctors only need to fill the heart rate column, to optimize the data storage. Each selected description will be ready as the standardized data that have been completed with the description with the smallest file size and will be directly stored in the database that could be easily recognized by the system. **Figure 3** shows the tele-ECG application that has been used for Makassar Telemedicine Program that provides services for 46 primary care centers distributed in urban, rural, including remote islands in East Indonesia.

7. Implementation of tele-ECG model in Makassar, Indonesia

The implementation of tele-ECG at more than 46 primary care centers in Indonesia has started in 2015, mainly in the South Sulawesi Province. Each primary care center provides tele-ECG services, not only for outpatient clinics but also for Emergency Department. The tele-ECG consultations were carried out for all patients with suspicion of heart disease, including acute coronary syndrome.

Makassar tele-ECG service runs routinely every day, with around 10,000 cardiac records have been transmitted in 4 years since its commencement. During the operation, every transmitted ECG record would get a quick response from the cardiology consultant. For the clinic services in primary care centers, on average, the ECG recordings were sent from morning to afternoon, and subsequently, the response and answers by the consultants would be delivered within 2–4 hours. In the case of acute or emergency settings, the operator will immediately notify the consultant for an immediate response. For normal ECG, the consultant only took 15 seconds to make the description of ECG. Meanwhile, for an abnormal ECG, the average time needed to describe the ECG was about 30–45 seconds. The tele-ECG answers can be immediately seen by the sender, i.e., nurse or GP at the primary care center, with available printable reading results when needed.

8. Data collection and measurement

Using an automated ECG equipment—the BTL-08 SD ECG (BTL Industries Ltd., Hertfordshire, United Kingdom)—trained primary care nurses collected patients' ECGs. The Hasanuddin University Hospital's analysis service center received the ECG files through the internet and stored them in the hospital's database. All of the ECG recordings were reviewed and examined by two cardiologists. Between August 2015 and February 2018, Makassar Telemedicine Service (MTS) received ~10,000 12-lead ECG recordings from patients in primary care.

In order to gather information on sociodemographic and clinical profiles (such as symptom, onset, prior disease, prior medication, anthropometric status, vital signs, and cardiovascular risk factors: hypertension, diabetes mellitus, current smoking, and family history of CVD), management and medications after tele-ECG, and GP's reasons for and satisfaction with tele-ECG consulting, a thorough questionnaire was developed. All participants had vital sign assessments, including blood pressure, heart rate, respiration rate, and axillary temperature, as well as anthropometrics, a routine physical examination, and ECG analysis. Manual measurements were taken

Classification	ECG patterns*	Total (n = 10,001)
Normal ECG	Normal sinus rhythm	7265 (72.6)
Ischemia	ST-elevation myocardial infarction	98 (1.0)
	Old myocardial infarction	548 (5.5)
	ST and/or T wave changes suggestive of MI	509 (5.1)
	Non-specific ST and/or T wave changes	99 (1.0)
Arrhythmia	Sinus bradycardia	892 (8.9)
	Sinus tachycardia	393 (3.9)
	Supraventricular tachycardia	11 (0.1)
	Atrial fibrillation	110 (1.1)
	Atrial flutter	9 (0.1)
	Atrial premature complexes	94 (0.9)
	Ventricular premature complexes	105 (1.0)
	Sino-atrial block	6 (0.1)
	Atrioventricular block	49 (0.5)
	Right bundle branch block	160 (1.6)
	Left bundle branch block	21 (0.2)
Structural change	Left atrial enlargement	45 (0.5)
	Right atrial enlargement	48 (0.5)
	Left ventricular hypertrophy	418 (4.2)
	Right ventricular hypertrophy	23 (0.2)
Others	Early repolarization	72 (0.7)
	Left axis deviation	184 (1.8)
	Right axis deviation	128 (1.3)
	Hyper/hypokalemia	37 (0.4)

**More than one ECG diagnosis per patient is possible.*
Values are n (%).res.
ECG = electrocardiogram; MI = myocardial infarction.

Table 1.
Interpretation of ECG recordings from Makassar telemedicine service.

for height, waist circumference, and body weight. Since these tests are typically not accessible at the primary care level, none of the laboratory tests—such as fasting plasma glucose, lipid profiles, and creatinine—was carried out. All these data were collected in a standardized database. The data were then converted into Excel format for further analysis in the SPSS statistical program for research purposes.

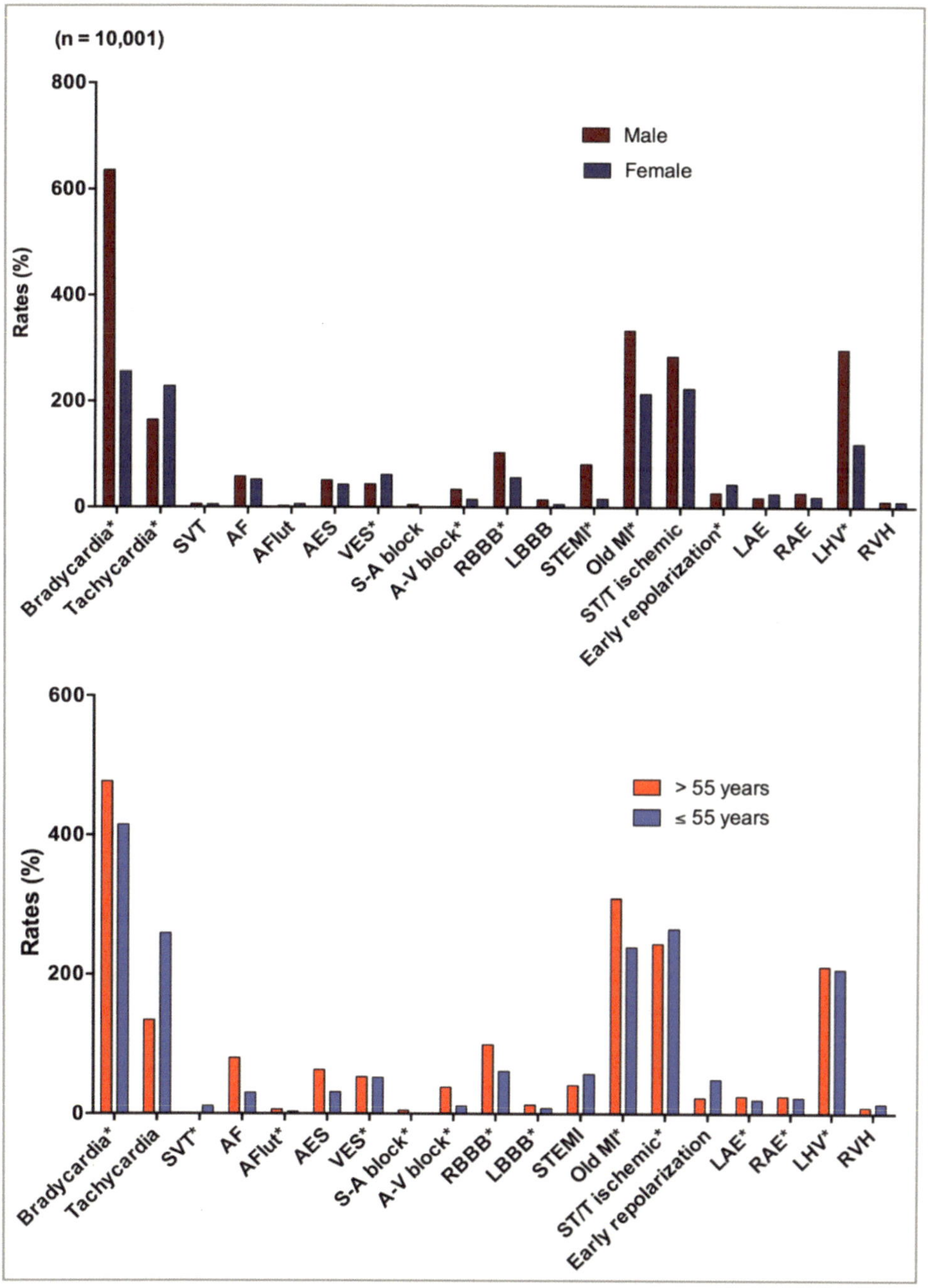

Figure 4.
Distribution of ECG abnormalities based on gender and age.

9. Implementation results: the first report from the tele-ECG program in Indonesia

A total of 10,001 ECG recordings were transferred to telemedicine program's analysis center at Hasanuddin University Hospital between 2015 and 2018. All ECG recordings were eligible for analysis. Around 73% of the overall ECG recordings were classified as normal. After ECG categorization, ischemia was discovered in 13% of cases, arrhythmia in 18%, and structural abnormalities in 5%. **Table 1** displays the analysis and distribution of all ECGs from the Makassar Telemedicine Program (n = 1001), while **Figure 4** shows the ECG abnormalities based on gender and age.

Our previous study shows that tele-ECG consulting was helpful to support GPs in primary care in making a quick decisions on patient management. Of 10,001 ECG screenings transmitted to the analysis center, 100% qualified for analysis.

Implementation of the tele-ECG program during these 4 years showed that the delivery process run smoothly, as there were always 5–10 tele-ECG recordings transmitted from several primary healthcare centers every working day. The succession of this implementation is supported by the local government provided the infrastructure; trained nurses and GPs who made the first screening and risk stratification; and immediate response of the expert, cardiologists to read and answer the teleconsultation. This fact showed a piece of robust evidence that the design and model of the tele-ECG program that prioritized the easiness for both the senders and readers and smooth internet connection had been successfully implemented in the archipelagic areas.

In view of cardiology services, 88 patients for whom hospital admission was advised, 72 (81.8%) were immediately referred within 48 hours following the tele-ECG consultation. Thus far, this tele-ECG program has been successfully carried out with two main purposes, healthcare services, and research, that ultimately help in improving patient outcomes.

SVT, supraventricular tachycardia; AF, atrial fibrillation; Aflut, Atrial Flutter; AES, atrial extra systole; VES, ventricular extra systole; S-A block, sinoatrial block; A-V block, atrioventricular block; RBBB, right bundle branch block; LBBB, left bundle branch block; STEMI, ST-elevation myocardial infarction; Old MI, old myocardial infarction; LAE, left atrial enlargement; RAE, right atrial enlargement; LVH, left ventricular hypertrophy; RVH, right ventricular hypertrophy.

10. Conclusions: philosophy of tele-ECG implementation

- Telemedicine program is about function, not sophistication. And thus, placed the tele-ECG program in the areas where it is needed the most.

- The main goal of telemedicine in archipelagic areas is not about healing the patients' disease, but beyond this, concern and sustainability.

- When technology is in hand, while the natural conditions are out of reach, then technology follows nature.

- The basis of telemedicine research is healthcare services, therefore, addressing the service function first and patients data would follow the way.

Acknowledgements

The participants in Makassar's primary care centers are warmly acknowledged for their willingness to take part in this tele-ECG program. We also thank the patients' advisors and family members for their participation and support. We appreciate Makassar City's municipal government's assistance in putting tele-ECG into daily practice. We also thank the employees and residents at Pusat Jantung Terpadu Makassar Cardiac Center for their contributions to the accomplishment of this telemedicine project. We acknowledge all research assistants, primary care nurses, cadres, and personnel that helped with data administration for this study.

Conflict of interest

The authors declare no conflict of interest.

Author details

Idar Mappangara[1*] and Andriany Qanitha[2]

1 Faculty of Medicine, Department of Cardiology and Vascular Medicine, Hasanuddin University, Makassar, Indonesia

2 Faculty of Medicine, Department of Cardiology and Vascular Medicine; Department of Physiology; Doctoral Study Program, Hasanuddin University, Makassar, Indonesia

*Address all correspondence to: idar.unhas@gmail.com

References

[1] Shrestha BM. Telemedicine and virtual health care during coronavirus disease pandemic. Journal of Nepal Medical Association. 2020;**58**:547-556

[2] World Health Organization. A health telematics policy - in support of WHO's health-for-all strategy for global health development

[3] World Health Organization. Implementing Telemedicine Services During COVID-19: Guiding Principles and Considerations for a Stepwise Approach. 2020. pp. 1-25. Available from: http://iris.wpro.who.int/handle/10665.1/14651

[4] Hsiao CH, Shiau CY, Liu YM, Chao MM, Lien CY, Chen CH, et al. Use of a rich internet application solution to present medical images. Journal of Digital Imaging. 2011;**24**:967-978

[5] Klabunde RE. Cardiac electrophysiology: Normal and ischemic ionic currents and the ECG. Advances in Physiology Education. 2017;**41**:29-37

[6] Mappangara I, Qanitha A, Uiterwaal CSPM, Henriques JPS, de Mol BAJM. Tele-ECG consulting and outcomes on primary care patients in a low-to-middle income population: The first experience from Makassar telemedicine program, Indonesia. BMC Family Practice. 2020;**21**:1-11

[7] Mboi N, Murty Surbakti I, Trihandini I, Elyazar I, Houston Smith K, Bahjuri Ali P, et al. On the road to universal health care in Indonesia, 1990-2016: A systematic analysis for the global burden of disease study 2016. The Lancet. 2018;**392**:581-591

[8] Horton R. Offline: Indonesia - Unravelling the mystery of a nation. The Lancet. 2016;**387**:830

[9] Cardiovascular Division & Health Services Research Centre. Reducing the burden of CVD in Indonesia: Evidence review. Newtown: The George Institute for Global Health; 2017

[10] Kementerian Kesehatan Republik Indonesia. Situasi kesehatan jantung. Pusat data dan informasi kementerian kesehatan Republik Indonesia. 2014:3

[11] Ministry of Health Republic of Indonesia. Riset Kesehatan Dasar (Riskesdas) 2013. Badan Penelitian dan Pengembangan Kesehatan Kementerian Kesehatan Republik Indonesia

[12] Binns C, Hokama T, Low WY. Island Health: Hope and challenges for public health. Asia-Pacific Journal of Public Health. 2010;**22**:19-24

[13] Myrick JG, Hendryx M. Health information source use and trust among a vulnerable rural disparities population. Journal of Rural Health. 2021;**37**:537-544

[14] Moore PT, O'Hare N, Walsh KP, Ward N, Conlon N. Objective video quality measure for application to tele-echocardiography. Medical and Biological Engineering and Computing. 2008;**46**:807-813

[15] Weisser G, Engelmann U, Ruggiero S, Runa A, Schröter A, Baur S, et al. Teleradiology applications with DICOM-e-mail. European Radiology. 2007;**17**:1331-1340

[16] Ling-ling W, Ni-ni R, Li-xin P, Gang W. Developing a DICOM middleware to implement ECG

conversion and viewing. Annual International Conference of the IEEE Engineering in Medicine and Biology – Proceedings. Vol. 7. 2005. pp. 6953-6956

[17] Bond RR, Finlay DD, Nugent CD, Moore G. A review of ECG storage formats. International Journal of Medical Informatics. 2011;**80**:681-697

[18] Hsieh JC, Lo HC. The clinical application of a PACS-dependent 12-lead ECG and image information system in E-medicine and telemedicine. Journal of Digital Imaging. 2010;**23**:501-513

Chapter 3

Low-cost Approaches to Follow-up Cardiac Patients in Low-Income Countries Using Public Data Networks

Rene Ivan Gonzalez-Fernandez, Margarita Mulet-Cartaya, Gisela Montes de Oca-Colina, Jorge Aguilera-Perez, Juan Dayron Lopez-Cardona and Jose Luis Hernandez-Caceres

Abstract

The main characteristics of three approaches to cardiac care using public data networks are presented. All efforts were addressed to get minimum-cost solutions for low-budget public health systems. The first solution was developed to follow-up arrhythmic patients between medical consultations, setting a more closed patient-physician relationship, and a daily recording of cardiac rhythm changes. It is based on a personal battery-powered device for one-channel ECG recording, minimizing electrode setting and operation complexity. An ECG recording taken daily allows a detailed analysis anytime without the patient's traveling to a health institution. A second solution was aimed at monitoring high-risk cardiac patients. A 24-h portable device capable of monitoring heart rate and sudden falls, typically associated with cardiac syncope, was developed. When any cardiac event or fall is detected, an urgent message is sent to relatives and the medical emergency care system asking for help. The third system implemented is oriented to the study of different cardiac parameters in people who suffer from heart disease or in those who are prone to suffering from it. Twelve-lead ECG is recorded periodically by each patient and trend graphics reflect ECG parameters strongly associated with cardiac disturbances, such as sudden death and ischemia. This approach allows the detection of the first troubling electrocardiographic deviations, making possible early medical intervention.

Keywords: telemedicine, cardiac home care, ECG processing, cardiac syncope identification, arrhythmia analysis, cardiac disturbance predictors

1. Introduction

For decades, heart disease has been the leading cause of death worldwide, according to periodic reports from the World Health Organization (WHO) [1, 2]. The high consumption of so-called junk food, sedentary lifestyle, smoking, and other conditions have driven humankind to this situation. Some years ago, heart disease as the leading cause of death was strongly associated with high-income countries, but nowadays it has been extended to medium and low-income countries, displacing infectious-contagious diseases. In poor countries, the situation becomes even more critical since their economies do not have sufficient resources to face the cost of therapies, medical devices, and high-qualified physicians to cover the population, so the public health system falls into crisis frequently.

The resting electrocardiogram (ECG) is worldwide the leading test to detect cardiac disorders; more than 100 million of ECGs are indicated in the United States annually [3]. For any surgery procedure, it is mandatory to check the cardiovascular status previously and for the rest ECG is the ideal test, since it is noninvasive, easy to perform, and highly standardized, offering significant information about the cardiovascular system status. Its interpretation is supported by more than 100 years of accumulated knowledge [4].

Devices and methods for automatic ECG acquisition and processing have greatly evolved, making it possible for this technology to be used efficiently after minimal training. In fact, several systems have been developed combining this kind of devices with public data networks, web applications, and the proper procedures allowing the implementation of telecardiology services [5–7]. However, new solutions emerge continuously because each region and country have needed a customizing process according to local requirements.

The authors of this chapter have developed solutions that provide health services aimed at the care of heart diseases, but these approaches could be extended to other chronic diseases. The solutions presented have the following in common:

- They are focused on the treatment of cardiac patients.
- Combine the use of public data networks with medical devices for personal or home use.
- They minimize the operating cost of the solution without sacrificing high performance and quality standards.

The authors hope the discussed topics will motivate other specialists to contribute to the continuous improvement of public health services, mainly in low-income countries that suffer from the most critical situations.

2. Follow-up of persons suffering from cardiac arrhythmia

Cardiac arrhythmia is a chronic disease, so persons suffering must visit their cardiologist periodically to check their condition and the medical treatment effectiveness; this is the traditional approach to follow-up persons suffering from chronic disease. The main disadvantage is that changes and disorders occurring between a visit to the cardiologist and the next one never been recorded or known by the cardiologist. Suddenly, no evidence of why the patient got worse after a visit to the cardiologist and died inexplicably, and this is a non-infrequent situation.

The proposal of the authors solves the described situation. The patients are trained to use a portable medical device and are able to acquire and transmit a one-channel ECG, enough for cardiac rhythm analysis purposes. The digital ECG is uploaded to a website in order to be processed, stored, and reviewed at any time by the cardiologist in charge of the studied person. This specialist indicates the frequency of ECG acquisition, maybe 2 or 3 days, and trend charts are generated with the data extracted from the stored signals. This approach provides an easy way to know what changes in the cardiac rhythm take place day by day, contributing to a very close patient-cardiologist relationship. Dynamically, medical treatment can be changed when an abnormal situation is detected. All the process contributes to minimize patient's discomfort and agglomerations at hospital centers since visits to cardiologist can be reduced.

2.1 The proposed solution

The proposed system enables ECG recording several times per day, so the patient's condition can be analyzed with a detailing level impossible to get with the traditional approach. Any change can be studied from its first manifestations. Another feature to remark on is the possibility to make changes in the medical treatment dynamically, only with a phone call after analyzing the ECGs stored in the system's database. In addition, by reducing the frequency of visits to the cardiologist, patients improve their comfort and agglomerations in hospitals are reduced.

The development of the proposed system was divided into three parts as follows:

- The ECG recorder: A portable medical device to acquire one-channel ECG and transfer digital samples using a Bluetooth channel.
- The Android terminal: An Android-based application to receive the digital ECG transmitted from the ECG recorder, store and upload it to the analysis station when connectivity is available.
- The analysis station: A web application to store, analyze, and display the ECGs and the information associated with them.

Each part will be explained in detail below. The proposed solution can be viewed as a three-layer system. A first layer for the acquisition of the ECG with the developed portable device, a second layer is based on an Android application to guarantee connectivity with the web, data integrity, and a third layer, the web level, where the transferred ECGs are stored and processed. The web application provides complementary tools to help cardiologists to study the evolution of each patient. A representation of the proposed solution is shown in **Figure 1**.

2.1.1 The ECG recorder

A battery-powered medical device was developed to digitize a bipolar ECG lead; the authors recommend to attach the electrodes as it was defined for lead II from the standard 12-lead ECG because it is the best approach to study cardiac rhythm disturbances.

The ECG recorder was designed as a low-cost solution, so commercial electronic components were used instead of ASIC, FPGA, and so on. However, surface montage electronic components were combined with a multilayer print circuit design to reduce the device size and improve its reliability. The ECG recorder description can be divided as follows:

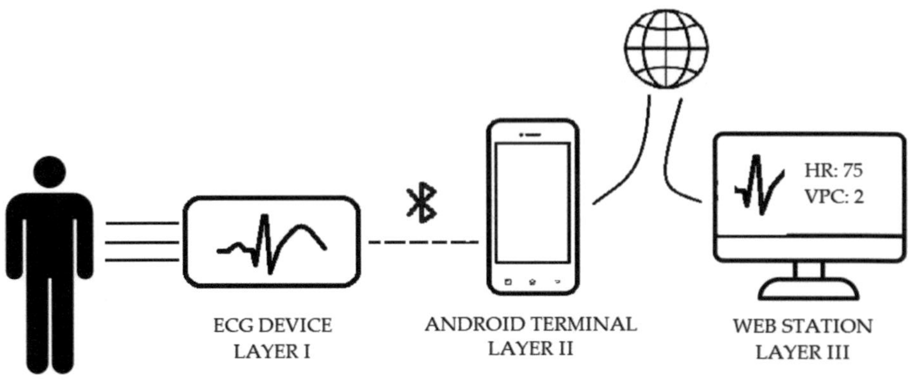

Figure 1.
The proposed three-layer system.

- The ECG amplifier: A low-noise one-channel ECG amplifier was designed to digitize a bipolar ECG lead characterized by its low power consumption. The amplifier design is based on the OPA4236 operational amplifier and the micro power single-supply INA826 instrumentation amplifier to get a very low power consumption, below 10 μA. The bandwidth is limited between 0.5 and 40 Hz to improve the signal quality and to keep the main ECG frequency components.

- The central processing unit: The MSP430F5529 microcontroller from Texas Instruments was selected as "the heart" of the ECG recorder; it is in charge of the control of the device functioning and all the computing tasks. This microcontroller is an ultralow-power component with a 16-bit RISC architecture and high-level integration. Several peripherals, such as serial ports, interrupt controllers, timers, memory, and A/D converter, are integrated into a single chip.

- The Bluetooth block: The first version was developed with the LMX9838 Bluetooth serial port module because it was mentioned as a standard by several electronic component manufacturers when the use of Bluetooth became widespread. This module is too expensive for our purpose, so a cheaper alternative was selected, it was the RN4678 module. This component provides a friendly and reliable solution for Bluetooth communication; the host communicates with the RN4678 sending commands interpreted and executed by a Bluetooth stack in charge of wireless bidirectional communication.

- The power unit: Two AAA NiMH batteries supply the required isolated voltage for the planned autonomy. A battery-charging circuit was not included to simplify the device and reduce its dimension, so batteries should be charged in any commercial charging station. A better solution will be a lithium polymer battery, not available in the market at the time when the design was developed.

ECG samples are acquired automatically when the ECG recorder is turned on; the sampling frequency always is set to 250 Hz. Bluetooth protocol is used to transmit digital samples to a mobile phone. Additional information about pacemaker spikes and electrode contact is transmitted too. A circuit for pacemaker spike identification was included in the ECG amplifiers; spike detection is based on signal slope analysis. Another circuit was designed to detect poor contact between the electrodes and the patient's skin; this process is very important because only one signal is available and its quality is very important for the intended use (**Figure 2**).

ECG samples, pacemaker information, and electrode status are packed and sent with a sync byte. The receiving, called the Android terminal (an app running on an Android-based mobile telephone) can identify the start of each packet and extract the information bits corresponding to ECG samples, electrode status, and pacemaker spike detection. ECG strip duration is set according to the study to be performed; a typical duration could be 3 min. When ECG transmission is finished, the MSP430F5529 microcontroller goes to "sleep mode" in order to minimize energy consumption. Only hardware interrupts generated by the keypad or the timer are able to wake the microcontroller.

2.1.2 The android terminal

This android application was programmed in Java language, but several other options are available nowadays; the same happens with the programming framework. The best choice of these items will strongly depend on the programmer's skills and will be determinant to shorten or delay the time to get the final solution.

The main features of this part of the proposed solution are the following:

- Device pairing: It is a mandatory process to set the Bluetooth link between the ECG recorder and the Android telephone. It is set for one time unless hardware changes or fails. It started with the mobile telephone.

- Bluetooth communication: The hardware components selected are fully compatible with this wireless communication standard, so a reliable channel is implemented. A user-level protocol was defined by the authors to guarantee a continuous data flow. ECG samples are transferred by blocks and information about electrode status and presence of pacemaker spikes is added. Control commands are included as head and tail for each block, contributing to easy synchronization.

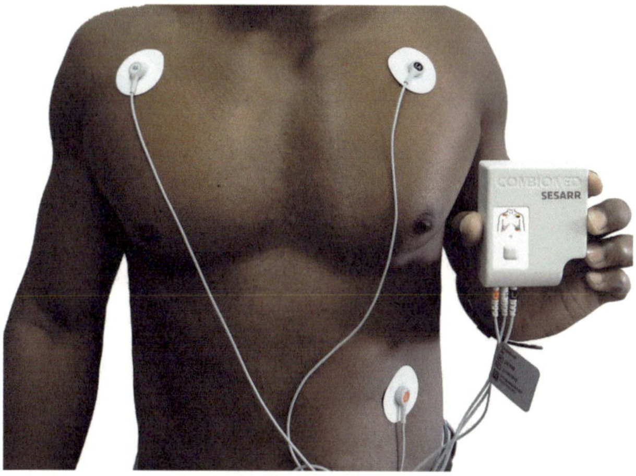

Figure 2.
The ECG recorder prototype.

- Database operations: MySQL was the database engine selected because of its compatibility with the SQL standard and its simplicity. The database to implement is not heavy or complex, so the selection is proper for the intended use. Addition, sorting, and querying are the most common operations in this application. The access is controlled by a password mechanism.

- ECG uploading: This feature considers that noncontinuous connectivity is a real possibility; accordingly, the proposed solution has been designed thinking in poor countries' conditions, where public communication networks are not as stable as the same service in First World countries. ECGs received from the recorder are stored in the Android terminal's database as a backup and are uploaded when connectivity is available using a secure HTTP protocol. The uploading process includes an encryption algorithm to avoid unauthorized personal data publication since it is mandatory in telemedicine systems [8].

2.1.3 The analysis station

This web application is the main part of the proposed solution because it enables cardiologists to analyze the status of any patient based on the collection of all signals captured by the ECG recorders and powerful graphic tools. Several parameters are computed as a complement of the stored digital ECG. A simple SQL database was implemented to store all general data, ECGs, and parameters. Tables and graphics are available to analyze the evolution of any patient, so cardiologists can evaluate the effectiveness of the drug treatment and make any necessary changes. Cardiologists' comments and treatment changes are stored in the database too. In summary, the analysis station provides the following features:

- User access control: A username and password mechanism are implemented to set a one-to-one relationship between cardiologists and their patients. Each cardiologist reviews ECG associated with his/her patients only.

- Trend charts of different electrocardiographic parameters: This kind of graphics represents parameter changes versus time, so cardiologist can observe when dangerous situations start their clinical manifestation. For instance, isolated heart rate changes are not dangerous, but it is so different when the change is observed continuously.

- Reports: Any table of graphics can be printed or stored as a PDF file. It is so useful to discuss any complex situation with other specialists or to create patient paper files.

- Export results: It is implemented to allow interoperability with other digital systems.

A simple way to appreciate the advantages of the proposed solution is the following example: A cardiologist instructs a patient to capture three ECGs daily with the ECG recorder (morning, afternoon, and night). After a month, the cardiologist has 90 ECGs of the specific patient and he/she can analyze in detail how it is influencing medical treatment in the disease studied. Following the traditional method of visits to the specialist, so much valuable information would never be accumulated. This is why it is said that the proposed system allows a much closer doctor-patient relationship.

Digital ECGs are processed at the analysis station to facilitate future software updating tasks. It is easier to update the web application only than to update each of the ECG recorder devices connected to the system or the Android app linked to each one.

2.1.4 ECG processing

ECG processing starts with digital filtering to remove or attenuate spurious signals. A FIR (finite impulse response) moving average filter proposed by Ligtenberg and Murat [8] was implemented. It was used by the authors in previous projects with good results; an attractive characteristic is that the filter is based on integer arithmetic only. The mathematical expression of the proposed filter is as follows:

$$y(k) = \frac{1}{K^2} \sum_{m=k-K+1}^{k} \sum_{n=m-K+1}^{m} x(n) - \frac{1}{L^2} \sum_{m=k-L+1}^{k} \sum_{n=m-L+1}^{m} x(n) \tag{1}$$

where x(n) is the input signal, y(k) is the output filtered signal, K, L are filter constants strongly associated with cut-off frequencies.

The authors have implemented a QRS complex detection based on an energy collector and two thresholds. The energy function is easy to implement because it is based on integer arithmetic; it is an important feature because the same function can be used for real time and offline applications with similar performances.

The energy function is defined as the sum of the squared differences of the samples corresponding to a preestablished time window previous to the studied sample. The windows width is set to 150 ms taking into count the width of ventricular beats which are prone to durations over 120 ms. Eq. (2) corresponds to the described energy collector.

$$y(k) = \frac{1}{N} \sum_{n=k-N+1}^{k} [x(n) - x(n-1)]^2 \tag{2}$$

where x(n) is the input signal, y(k) is the energy function.

The energy function is combined with two thresholds. The first one is used to detect high-energy peaks and the second threshold is applied to a rough onset and offset identification for each QRS complex. R waves are identified as the wave including the most positive peaks within each QRS complex, so a peak detection algorithm is applied after the onset and offset events were detected.

RR intervals are computed after the identification of all R wave's peaks as the difference between two consecutive peaks. Each cardiac beat is classified as premature or not premature according to their previous RR interval duration. An ECG strip is classified as "arrhythmic" if more than 10% of QRS detected gets into this classification. This percentage should be defined at the Android terminal setup and cardiologists can be modified according to the patients.

The information associated with each digital ECG is stored in a temporary database and uploaded to a sHTTP server. The temporary mobile telephone database can be very useful when public data network is out of service for a prolonged period due to natural disasters, army conflicts, and similar situations. When public data networks are not available, ECG can be reviewed in a limited framework.

The system operation can be summarized as follows:

1. Patients are enrolled in the system. Each patient receives the user guide, the ECG recorder (including patient cable and electrodes), and the Android terminal is installed on his phone.

2. The cardiologist explains to the patient his/her role in the system and an ECG strip is acquired as patient training.

3. The patient prepares his skin, by means of a light cleaning, and attaches the electrodes in the appropriate positions to acquire lead II unless the cardiologist indicates another configuration of electrodes.

4. The incoming digital ECG is filtered; the QRS complexes are detected and classified; and heart rate and ectopic beat rate are computed. All data are stored in a database and uploaded to sHTTP server.

5. The analysis station checks the sHTTP server periodically looking for new ECG data files. When new files are detected, all the uploaded information is into a database.

6. The cardiologists log in to the analysis station to study any patient. Each cardiologist can study his patients only. Arrhythmic evolution is analyzed and the treatment is corrected if necessary.

2.2 Results and discussion

Five ECG recorder prototypes have been tested according to the IEC 60601-2-47 standard and all results were successful. The proposed device is not a pure ambulatory medical device, but the IEC 60601-2-47 standard is suitable for its evaluation. Some of the most highlighted results are shown in **Table 1**.

The proposed device is safe for patients, according to the test results, following the IEC 60601-2-47 standard requirements.

The android terminal application was fully tested. The Bluetooth communication was checked with 200 simulated 3 min ECG strips with different heart rates: 60, 80, 120, and 150 beats per minute. These strips were acquired with three ECG recorders wireless connected to a mobile phone running the proposed Android terminal. This

Test	Result
Dynamic input range	5 mV
Input impedance	Greater than 2.5 MΩ
Maximum DC input level	320 mV
Internal noise	Less than 25 μV
Patient auxiliary current	Less than 0.01 mA
Setting time	Less than 3 s
Common mode reject ratio	Greater than 90 dB
IEC 60601-1 classification	Class I, BF type

Table 1.
Some results from technical tests.

test passed without errors, and the signals received by the Android terminal were identical to the original simulated ECGs. Also, the communication process was never aborted by errors.

The digital filter performance has been published in previous papers, so the authors do not consider necessary new evaluation [9]. A similar situation happens with the QRS detection process based on the previous experiences of the authors [9, 10]. Nevertheless, the authors considered it useful for the readers to show the performance when the algorithm was tested with the MIT-BIH arrhythmia database; results are shown in **Table 2**.

Thus, the performance of the QRS complex detection algorithm is enough for the intended use. The MIT-BIH arrhythmia database is a golden reference to test this kind of algorithm.

All the features of the proposed Android terminal have been tested with a significant amount of ECG strips. The performance of the implemented Bluetooth link has

Record	QRS	Detected	Sensitivity (%)	Record	QRS	Detected	Sensitivity (%)
100	2273	2273	100.00	201	1963	1960	99.85
101	1863	1861	99.89	202	2136	2127	99.58
102	2187	2160	98.77	203	2980	2963	99.43
103	2084	2084	100.00	205	2656	2624	98.80
104	2229	2220	99.60	207	1860	1833	98.55
105	2572	2549	99.11	208	2955	2933	99.26
106	2027	2007	99.01	209	3005	2996	99.70
107	2137	2120	99.20	210	2650	2631	99.28
108	1762	1741	98.81	212	2748	2746	99.93
109	2532	2507	99.01	213	3251	3220	99.05
111	2124	2111	99.39	214	2262	2241	99.07
112	2539	2538	99.96	215	3363	3360	99.91
113	1795	1794	99.94	217	2208	2177	98.60
114	1877	1860	99.09	219	2154	2136	99.16
115	1953	1951	99.90	220	2048	2046	99.90
116	2412	2398	99.42	221	2427	2407	99.18
117	1535	1520	99.02	222	2483	2466	99.32
118	2278	2253	98.90	223	2605	2581	99.08
119	1987	1981	99.70	228	2053	2018	98.30
121	1863	1861	99.89	230	2256	2253	99.87
122	2476	2475	99.96	231	1571	1568	99.81
123	1518	1516	99.87	232	1780	1772	99.55
124	1619	1592	98.33	233	3079	3036	98.60
200	2601	2576	99.04	234	2753	2750	99.89

Table 2.
Results with 12 ECG strips from MIT-BIH database.

been stable; no user-level errors have been detected. QRS complex detection algorithm was tested with MIT-BIH arrhythmia database, an international standard for this purpose, and the sensitivity was high, this result is enough for the intended use.

As has been seen, a full version of the proposed solution has been tested with satisfactory results. The ECG recorder safety meets the requirements set by the IEC 60601-1 standard for this kind of medical technology. The functioning of the system has been tested in stressing conditions without failures, demonstrating the robustness of the proposed solution.

The proposed system looks like a useful tool to study arrhythmic patient progression using existing data networks, mainly mobile telephone networks. Other chronic diseases can be studied following the same philosophy.

3. Cardiac monitoring of high-risk persons

Those persons who are subjected to high stress as part of their daily activities and do not have healthy lifestyle habits are prone to suffer from serious and sudden cardiovascular disorders, whose main manifestations are high blood pressure, malignant cardiac arrhythmia events, and acute myocardial infarctions. This kind of person needs continuous cardiac monitoring to detect dangerous changes since their beginning. Implanted cardiac loop recorders could be a solution for persons suffering from this situation, but these devices and the associated surgery procedure are expensive [11]. Besides, the risk associated with any surgery is always present.

An alternative without surgical risk and much cheaper would be the development of a device capable of monitoring the heart rhythm and transferring the digital signal to a remote central station when any dangerous change is detected from the analyzed person. For this data transfer, the existing public mobile data network in the country would be useful. The authors of this chapter focused their efforts on this kind of solution and present a proposal.

3.1 Proposal for out-of-hospital cardiac monitoring

We have developed a cardiac telemonitoring system as part of a larger telecardiology system with other final applications. The proposed system is composed of connected two parts using the mobile data network:

- ECG recorder: It is a small battery-powered device able to acquire and process one ECG channel in real time. When a dangerous event is detected, an ECG strip is transferred to the response central station and the device waits for instructions for the analyzed person about what to do. Several different indications can be sent, "relax and wait for an ambulance," "relax and send an ECG strip in 10 min" or person's intervention is not required because the process starts due to a false positive alarm.

- Response central station: A set of personal computers are connected as a local network linked to the public mobile data network to keep available to receive any request from the recorders integrated into the proposed system. A group of medical specialists is in charge of responding to incoming requests. When a help request is received, the ECG strip, some electrocardiographic parameters, and GPS location are displayed on a personal computer screen and an acoustic message is activated. A specialist analyzes the information and send the proper response, all the process (arriving time, delay to response, and specialist in charge) is stored in a database because this information is useful to optimize the system's performance. The response central station works together with the available ambulances to assign the closest one to the person who requires it.

The target of the ECG recorder design was to minimize the cost without decreasing its reliability. Besides, the device should be user-friendly, safe, and resistant to mechanical impacts. The device is composed of the following blocks:

- The ECG amplifier: It is a two-channel ECG amplifier characterized by its low power consumption, measured below 10 μA. The LT1496 operational amplifier and the micro power single-supply INA321 instrumentation amplifier are the main components of the proposed amplifier. The bandwidth is limited between 1 and 30 Hz in order to improve the signal quality and to keep the ECG frequency components associated with the intended use. The second ECG channel is used as a backup because electrode failures are common in long-term ambulatory ECG monitoring devices, so the channel with the best signal-to-noise ratio is used to extract cardiac rhythm information.

- The processing unit: The MSP430F149 microcontroller from Texas Instrument was selected as the processing unit. It is an ultralow-power and a highly integrated microcontroller with a 16-bit RISC architecture. Several peripherals, such as serial ports, timers, memory, and A/D converter, and an interrupt request controller, are integrated into a single chip. Also, a very large collection of application notes and examples of applications with this microcontroller are available, making easy its use in new products.

- The wireless communication module: The SIM928A module was selected for this purpose; it is a module that integrates into a single container GSM/GPRS and GPS standards. The mobile phone section is GSM/GPRS type and can operate in the most common bands. In terms of connectivity, this module has two UARTs for serial communication and also integrates TCP/IP functionality and extended AT commands to manage it. Its compact dimensions (30 × 30 × 3 mm), allow to develop very compact devices, such as trackers.

- The display unit: The LCD display used is the model GF5123FBWBF from crystal clear technology; its graphic resolution is 128 × 64 dots. The intended use is to show several data as part of the user interface and to check signal quality using its graphic capabilities. Also, messages from the response central station are displayed if patient cooperation is required.

- The keypad: Setup data is introduced using this soft-touch keypad. It is composed of five keys and is water-protected to avoid damage caused by spilled liquids.

- The power unit: The required isolated voltage is supplied by two NiMH batteries, which are recharged in a charging station when the device is not in use. It is recommended to move to lithium polymer technology to increase the device's autonomy (**Figure 3**).

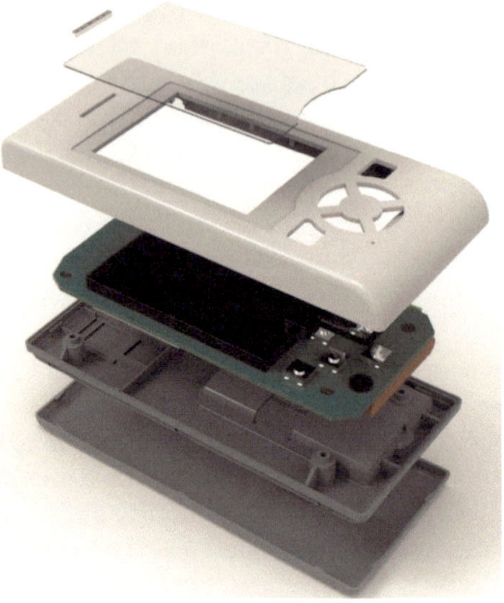

Figure 3.
Representation of the ECG recorder design.

The electronic design of the ECG recorder was made on a single printed circuit board; the LCD display and the GSM modem are connected to this board using board-to-board connectors. This design approach is robust against severe mechanical impacts and guarantees continuous functioning.

Two bipolar ECG leads are analyzed in real time to detect dangerous events, such as severe cardiac rhythm disturbances and pronounced ST-segment deviations. Since the cardiac patient's conditions are known a priori, the location of the electrodes can be adjusted to capture the ST-segment deviation in a given plane. It should not be forgotten that the heart is a three-dimensional organ and ST-segment deviations can manifest differently in different planes. However, the heart rhythm is unique and can be observed in the same way in any lead, although lead II is preferred due to its coincidence with the ventricular depolarization main vector. The ECG analysis algorithm can be divided as follows: ECG acquisition, QRS-complex detection, QRS-complex classification, ST-segment deviation measurement, and communication.

ECG samples are acquired from two bipolar channels simultaneously using s sampling rate of 250 Hz, enough according to the sampling theorem [12]. A single channel could seem enough, but a second channel is used as a backup because it is known electrode contact is prone to failures in long-term ambulatory monitoring systems, so a good approach is to acquire two channels and select for cardiac rhythm analysis the one with the best signal-to-noise ratio. Also, the two channels provide a better approach to the ST-segment deviation analysis.

The digital ECG is smoothed using a Hanning filter and the energy function is computed sample-by-sample for each channel according to Eq. (2) previously shown.

The QRS-complex detection process is based on the energy collector function computing and two thresholds. The first one is set as 20% of the maximum value of energy and it is used to identify high-energy signal segments. It is known that QRS complexes are integrated by high-energy components. The second threshold is used to set a rough identification of the onset and offset for each QRS complex; it is set as 5% of the maximum energy value. The position of these events is refined using a derivative function and each QRS complex width is computed; the QRS complex candidates should reach a minimum duration (30 ms). The mean RR interval duration is updated when a new QRS complex is detected because its previous RR interval is calculated. A baseline estimation for each QRS complex is set as the mean value of the samples associated with 20 ms before the complex onset. The average heart rate is updated every 10 s.

The proposed system is focused on long-term real-time ambulatory monitoring, a much more complex scenario than the first explained system. This is the reason for introducing a change in the energy function. Instead of using a simple signal slope calculation, the authors introduce the Teager operator as the basis to obtain the signal energy.

The Teager operator is a nonlinear operator that mainly shows the frequency and instantaneous changes of the signal amplitude and is very sensitive to subtle changes. Although the Teager operator was first proposed for modeling nonlinear speech signals, it was later widely applied in ECG and EEG research [13]. Its expression is as follows:

$$TO(x[n]) = x^2[n] - (x[n-1] * x[n+1]) \tag{3}$$

where TO is the Teager operator, x[n] is the input signal.

Once the QRS complexes have been detected, they are classified to group them as normal (NB), premature (PB), and unclassified. This process is important for the measurement of ST-segment deviation, it is only measured in normal complexes, and for calculating the premature beats rate, which can alert about serious ventricular disorders. To facilitate the execution of these tasks in real time, the criteria to be used must be simple without losing effectiveness. The defined criteria were the following:

- A normal beat must be preceded by an RR interval whose duration is greater than 80% of the average duration of previously measured intervals of this type and less than 110% of it.

- The width of a normal QRS complex has to be greater than 85% of the average value of this variable for the previously detected complexes and less than 110% of it.

- A premature beat must be aberrant and its duration must be greater than 120% of the average value of this parameter for the previously detected QRS complexes.

- The RR interval preceding a premature beat (PB) must be short and this concept is expressed as 80% of the average duration of the previously measured RR intervals.

- The duration of RR interval previous to a premature beat (PB) must be less than 80% of the average duration of this interval.

The premature beats rate is updated every 10 s. Unclassified beats are not studied.

The ST-segment deviation is defined as the difference in voltage between the sample place 80 ms after the QRS complex onset and the baseline estimation for the studied complex (**Figure 4**).

When the ECG recorder is turned on and configured, a first information block is transmitted to the response central station in order to open a patient profile. This block includes the following information:

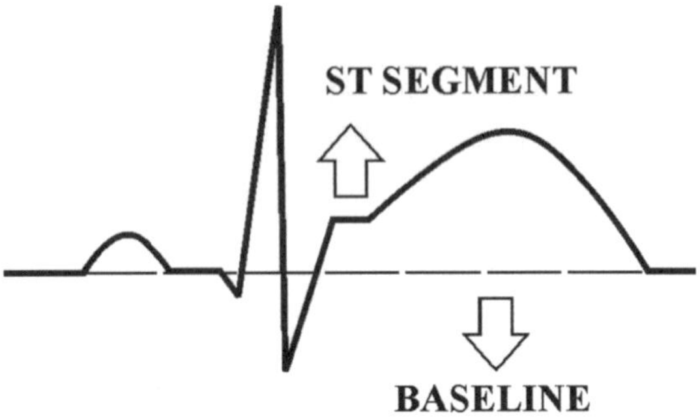

Figure 4.
ST-segment deviation.

- Device identification
- Sampling rate
- Amplitude resolution
- Channel quantity
- Studied variables (ST-segment deviation, heart rate, etc.) and their normality limits

The response central station responds with a block known as "echo block." If the ECG recorder requesting to be recognized is correctly identified, an echo block identical to the one sent by the ECG recorder is transmitted. If an error occurs and the ECG recorder is not properly identified, the response central station does not send a response block. The ECG recorder tries the connection three times before reporting the error on its screen so that the specialized personnel can take some action to solve this technical problem.

Since the ECG recorder is turned on; it will analyze the ECG in real time to transmit signal segments to the TCS when any electrocardiographic event reflecting a dangerous condition is detected or when the studied subject decides to send an ECG segment because he is feeling discomfort. Also, ECG segments can be sent periodically if the device is configured for this purpose.

Dangerous events that can be identified by the ECG recorder are marked tachycardia and bradycardia, high premature beats rate, and significant ST-segment deviations. The information is transmitted in blocks composed of a header that identifies the type of block, a body that contains the ECG samples, and a tail containing a checksum code to validate data integrity.

An identification block is sent to start the communication with the TCS. The transmitted ECG strip could be split into several signal blocks and, in the end, a final block is transmitted, including the block quantity transmitted. The ECG recorder will wait for an answer, which will be displayed if patient's cooperation is required.

3.2 Implementation results

Five ECG recorder prototypes were manufactured and tested.

The developed real time ECG processing method has been tested with 25 min ECGs, including eight ECGs with premature beats, from a Holter system. The signals were analyzed by two highly-qualified cardiologists with more than 20 year of experience in analyzing ECG strips. They were helped by a Windows application, developed by the authors of this document, which allowed them to carry out an exhaustive analysis of the digitized ECGs. These cardiologists were not aware of the method outcomes in order to perform a blind evaluation. The opinions and conclusions of the specialists were the golden rule to test the method. The evaluation results can be summarized in **Table 3**.

As can be seen in **Table 3**, all the QRS complexes present in the analyzed signals were detected. This result is remarkable because it is the basis for reliable ECG analysis.

It should not be forgotten that all processing is done in real time on a battery-powered device, so a vital requirement is low power consumption to ensure the expected runtime. For this reason, a trade-off between the simplicity of the rules for classifying QRS complexes and their effectiveness must also be achieved. Complex calculations imply high energy consumption.

The set rules for the QRS complexes classification are simple, and based on low-complexity computational operations. Despite this, they have demonstrated high effectiveness with more than 96% of identified premature complexes. Only a small number of normal QRS complexes were misclassified, but this flaw does not affect the intended use of this solution. The main objective is the early detection of cardiac events associated with ventricular disorders and the results obtained are satisfactory. It should be noted that a premature QRS complex was never considered normal, although some of them were identified as unclassified beats (UB).

The ST-measurement algorithm was not evaluated because it was not implemented for the ECG recorder's first version. However, the algorithm was implemented in order to evaluate the real-time performance of the proposed method.

Communication with the response central station was set under the following conditions: more than two premature beats in 10 s; heart rate value over 100 beat per second (bpm) or heart rate value below 60 bpm.

To test the communication process, 40 ECG strips were transferred and these operations were always successful. The signals received at the response central station were compared, sample by sample, with the originally transmitted signal. A graphic program was used for this test and remarkable differences were not observed. Also, communication never was unexpectedly, and the received signals were not corrupted by noise or distortions. These results confirm that the communication process was effective.

The proposed system seems a useful monitoring tool for patients prone to suffer sudden heart attacks. Also, it could be useful for long-term ECG studies.

Test	Result
QRS complexes studied	7268
QRS complexes detected	7268 (100%)
Normal QRS complexes	6993
Normal QRS well-classified	6830 (97.67%)
Ventricular QRS complexes	275
Ventricular QRS well-classified	266 (96.73%)

Table 3.
Global results of the proposed method for real time ECG analysis.

4. A tool for primary and secondary cardiac disease prevention in the community

It is internationally recognized that all public health systems should focus their efforts and resources on the prevention of chronic diseases, giving top priority to health services related to this purpose [14]. In the particular case of heart disease, the leading cause of death worldwide, the international scientific community accepts that there are certain electrocardiographic parameters strongly related to the prediction of severe cardiac disorders. Based on this criterion, it is proposed that if these parameters are long-term studied; it is possible to predict cardiovascular system complications and take therapeutic actions before they manifest.

Early detection of heart disease ensures that medical treatment is less aggressive and more effective than if the disease progresses to more advanced stages. This is the reason why several multidisciplinary groups of researchers are working to develop tools and strategies for the primary and secondary prevention of heart disease. Primary prevention means medical attention for people who are prone to develop heart disease because of their lifestyle or genetic facts, even before they get sick. These people must learn to improve their lifestyle (eliminating tobacco, proper nutrition, fitness, etc.), but it is also feasible to study them periodically to identify any change toward morbidity from its first manifestations. When a person has already had a heart attack, the medical procedure is to enter that person into a cardiac rehabilitation program. Secondary prevention focuses on inducing healthy lifestyles and regular screening for any early signs of another attack. The study of the evolution of different electrocardiographic parameters can contribute decisively to avoiding a new heart attack.

Resting ECG is an inexpensive cardiac test that provides valuable information for implementing the approaches described above.

The aim of this section is to present and discuss a system designed for the implementation of primary and secondary prevention of heart disease in the community. The periodic study of a group of electrocardiographic parameters is intended to evaluate their evolution and thus predict the onset of severe cardiac disorders. This study is focused on subjects who have already had a heart attack or who are prone to one.

4.1 How to help prevent cardiac diseases?

The proposed system is composed of two main elements: a portable device for rest ECG acquisition, henceforth, recorder and Windows-compatible software, called a. The designer team's aim was a low-cost device able to get a high-quality rest ECG and ready to be used anywhere, without special requirements. Besides, the proposed system will be addressed to the community and the neighborhood, so it should be friendly for the users, the family doctors, and nurses or paramedics.

4.2 The recorder

These recorders are based on an ARM9 microprocessor operating at a frequency of 400 MHz; they have the following features:

- Graphic LCD with touch screen interface
- Soft keypad

DOI: http://dx.doi.org/10.5772/intechopen.108222

- USB interface
- Embedded modem with TCP/IP stack
- Eight-channel ECG amplifier
- SD memory
- NiMH battery-pack
- Medical grade's power supply

The described hardware is enough for the intended use, but the cost could be reduced using alternatives available in the single-board computer market currently.

The multichannel ECG amplifier is dedicated to acquire and adequate the electrocardiographic signals generated by the patient. These analog signals are converted to digital values at a sampling rate of 500 Hz [12] (**Figure 5**).

The main features of the ECG multichannel amplifier are described below. An analog bandpass filter was implemented to limit the frequency spectrum of the signals between 0.05 and 100 Hz according to the requirements of the IEC 60601-2-25 standard. Each amplifier channel is protected against defibrillator discharge with 10 kΩ resistors. A classic right leg circuit for improved common mode rejection ratio was included as part of the amplifier [3]. Pacemaker spike detection is based on lead II; the signal at the output of the corresponding instrumentation amplifier is used to detect the spikes; and this signal is connected to the input of a filter capable of generating a pulse every time a spike is detected, while the rest of the time it has a zero as output.

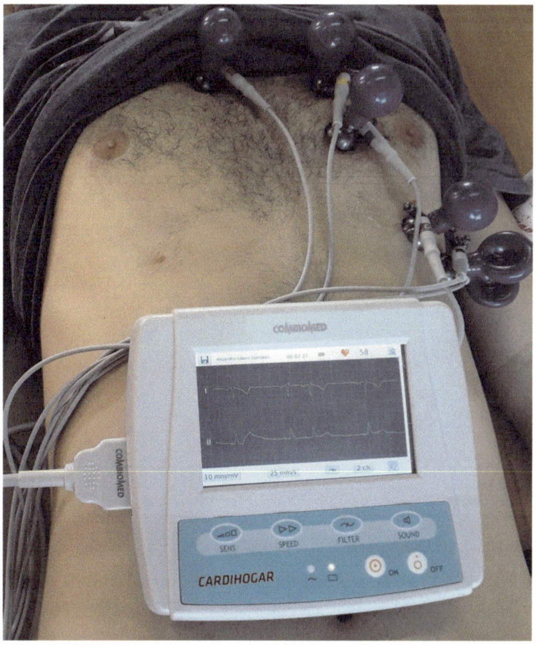

Figure 5.
View of the ECG recorder.

Another circuit called "trace recovery" is implemented to minimize the required time to recover the reference level when an electrode contact fails and any amplifier is saturated.

The eight independent leads (I, II, V1, V2, V3, V4, V5, and V6) are simultaneously digitized at a rate of 500 Hz with a 12-bit A/D converter; the LSB value is 3.15 microvolts. Leads III, aVR, aVL, and aVF are not implemented in the ECG amplifier because they can be derived from classical expressions when leads I and II are acquired simultaneously.

When signals from the eight channels have been acquired, two digital filters are applied. A notch filter is used to reject the 60 Hz component and a moving average type FIR filter is used to improve signal quality, minimizing noise and removing baseline wandering.

QRS complexes are detected in real time to calculate the heart rate when the ECG is acquired. A function of spatial velocity (FSV) is the basis for this process. This auxiliary function makes so easy to identify the signal segments associated with the QRS complexes [4].

$$FSV(k) = \sum_{i=1}^{C} [x(i,\ k) - x(i,\ k-1)]^2 \tag{4}$$

where FSV(k) is the Function of spatial velocity, x(i, k) is the ECG sample for lead i, C is the number of simultaneous leads.

As it is classic in the resting ECG devices, the electrocardiographic signals are acquired for 10 s and subsequently processed to extract the value of all the variables studied, more than 220 variables in each signal studied. However, the ECG is acquired without specifying when it will be analyzed; the operator is the one who decides when he wants the last 10 s of the ECG to be analyzed. While this process is going on, before it is analyzed in ECG, the device keeps calculating the heart rate in real time and updating its value on the screen every 10 s.

When the operator presses the proper button to start the ECG analysis, the signal acquisition process stops, and the ECG is analyzed automatically. More than 220 variables are calculated, and the process takes about 3 s. All this information is stored on the device. Computed variables can be grouped as follows:

- Amplitude and duration of P, P′, Q, R, S, R', and T waves.
- ST-segment deviation at the J point, the middle, and the end of the segment.
- PR, QT, and QRS interval widths.
- QT interval spatial dispersion.
- Corrected QT interval.
- Time of ventricular activation.

The recorder works as a data logger. For each ECG acquired, the recorder stores general patient data, the ECG (12 leads for 10 s), and measurements in internal memory where it maintains a database. This information is encrypted to guarantee its confidentiality. Data can be transferred to a computer using a USB connection.

Data and signals are displayed on the recorder's screen; it is a liquid crystal display (LCD) with a resolution of 800 × 600 pixels and colors. This peripheral greatly facilitates the interface with the operator. A flat, soft-key keyboard complements the operator interface while making cleanup easy.

In an emergency, the recorders can be connected to a telecardiology system to request specialized help. The recorder can send a digital ECG and receive guidance on the actions to take on the patient suffering from dangerous disturbances. The integrated modem is used to establish the connection using the traditional telephone network or using a TCP/IP stack.

4.3 The analyzer

The analyzer is a Windows application running on a personal computer with sufficient resources to store all information associated with each patient enrolled in the proposed system. **Figure 6** shows an ECG from a patient and a list, on the left extreme of the screen, of the acquired ECGs. The system language is configured as Spanish. Other languages may also be incorporated.

The physicians use a graphical interface to evaluate patient ECGs; they can see the ECG one by one or they can study the trend of different parameters and thus detect the first signs of a heart disorder. Also, they can upload complex ECGs to a web application, called "The Expert," looking for a second specialized opinion before taking decisions. The parameters studied are:

- Cornell and Sokolow Indexes: These indices are strongly associated with ventricular hypertrophy. They are computed for each ECG and their trend is represented in a proper chart. The aim of the long-term analysis of these indices is the early detection of a ventricular dilation process because this process appears at the beginning of ventricular hypertrophy. Medical intervention at the beginning of this ventricular disturbance could delay its negative effects or even avoid them.

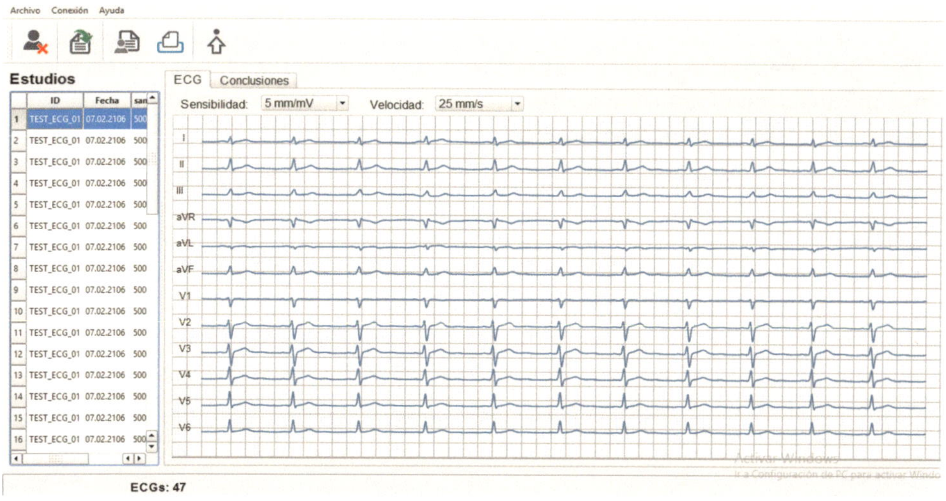

Figure 6.
ECG from a patient enrolled in the proposed system.

- QT interval spatial dispersion: Reported as an indicator to predict the onset of malignant arrhythmias [15]. Its analysis is a powerful surveillance tool for persons suffering from ventricular arrhythmias. A long-term study of QT interval dispersion for a patient could alert the family doctor about a forthcoming dangerous ventricular arrhythmic event; this kind of cardiac disturbance can provoke death or major cardiac damage. The proper analysis of the QT interval spatial dispersion using a trend chart constructed with big ECG data is a powerful tool for health services focused on cardiac care.

- Selvester scoring: This punctuation system assigns points according to criteria based on the amplitude and duration of waves of the QRS complexes. The accumulated points are proportional to the heart area damaged by a heart attack; it has been tested by taking autopsy data as a reference [16].

The proposed system studies the trend of the parameters mentioned above. Isolated values can be affected by different factors, while the tendency of a collection of values will indicate its behavior over time. All data associated with each study is displayed on the same screen to facilitate the analysis without continuous window changing.

4.4 Results and discussion

Five prototypes have been manufactured and tested; they have successfully passed parametric tests and electrical safety tests established in IEC 60601-2-25 for rest ECG devices with automatic wave measurement capabilities. Some of the main results of these tests, from the hardware point of view, are summarized in **Table 4**; it is impossible to show all of them because of the available space for the present document.

The obtained results meet the IEC 60601-1-25 requirements, so it is possible to affirm that the implemented electronic design solutions used in this device have been effective and according to the state-of-the-art. The software developed for ECG processing has been evaluated with CSE and CTS databases according to the same IEC standard [2]. For all studied variables, the maximum permissible error in measuring an ECG event has not been exceeded. Some of the results are shown in **Table 5**.

The QRS-detection algorithm was full-effective, and all the QRS complexes present in the analyzed ECGs were identified; all these signals are from the CTS and CSE databases, considered as an international standard. This result is very promising,

Parameter	Result
Frequency response	0.05–100 Hz
Accuracy and stability of the sensitivity	Less than ±5%
Intrinsic channel noise	Less than 30 μV
Common mode rejection ratio	Greater than 90 dB
Patient auxiliary current	Less than 50 μA
Permanent leakage current	Less than 300 μA
Classification according to IEC	Class 1, type CF

Table 4.
Main results of parametric tests.

Interval	Mean error (ms)	Standard Deviation (ms)
P wave	7.02	6.73
PQ interval	6.88	6.91
QRS complex	4.02	5.48
QT interval	8.17	5.12

Table 5.
Mean differences and standard deviations for global intervals on analytical ECGs.

although it can change a little under extreme-noisy conditions, so it is strongly recommended to take care to minimize noise presence.

When the accuracy of amplitude measurements within the QRS complex was analyzed, automatic measurements never deviated from the reference more than 25 microvolts for amplitudes lower than 500 microvolts or higher than 5% for amplitudes greater than 500 microvolts. This behavior meets the IEC standard requirements.

The full system has also been preliminarily tested with simulated signals and volunteers. The performance has been stable and there were no recorders out of order, software malfunctions, or unexpected errors. The proposed system has been completed with satisfactory results. All the IEC tests have passed successfully.

The analyzer works properly and is a friendly application. Five experienced cardiologists confirmed this criterion after several work sessions. By combining the available analysis tools and data, cardiologists can get new results unreachable using the traditional approaches. The proposed system seems a useful tool for cardiac disease prevention approach at the community level.

5. Final considerations

The three solutions described in this chapter are aimed at caring for subjects suffering from or prone to cardiac disorders. Two of these solutions are based on medical devices for personal use and the third is a system for the care of subjects in the community, in the environment in which they carry out their daily activities, based on the standard 12-lead ECG. In all solutions, public data networks are used to exchange information without requiring special services, so the cost is minimized for this concept.

Chronic diseases were associated with countries with high industrial development, while low-income countries were more linked with non-chronic diseases, such as dengue, diarrhea, and others. This situation has changed in recent years because of several factors and chronic diseases have reached an equal impact on all countries, regardless of their economic development. The great difference lies in the economic resources available to implement public health policies, while in developed countries the necessary resources are available, the health systems of underdeveloped countries are unable to serve the entire population due to their economic and financial limitations. The use of telemedicine, based on public data networks, can be a powerful tool to expand health services to everyone.

Table 6 summarizes some of the characteristics of the proposed solutions, showing the elements they have in common and their differences.

It should be noted that the three solutions have been developed in full adherence to the safety and performance requirements established in the IEC standards

Solution	Intended use	Basic standard	ECG channels	Basic operation mode
1	Arrhythmia follow-up	IEC 60601-2-47	1	Off-line
2	Ambulatory monitoring	IEC 60601-2-47	2	Real time
3	Disturbance prediction	IEC 60601-2-25	8	Off-line

Table 6.
Main characteristics of the proposed solutions.

(International Electrotechnical Commission), accepted as international standards and compatible with other similar institutions, such as FDA (Food and Drug Administration) and Japanese regulatory documents. Another aspect to highlight is the multidisciplinary teamwork for the development of the proposed solutions. The scientific level required for this software, mechanical, and electronic solutions was combined with the theoretical knowledge and practical experience of high-qualified cardiologists with more than 20 years dedicated to clinical services in their specialty, who provided valuable criteria for the implementation of the necessary features and for the evaluation of the proposed systems in real conditions of use.

One-channel and two-channel devices were developed to analyze cardiac rhythm disturbances; one solution focused on following up arrhythmic disease and the other for real time surveillance purposes to detect dangerous events immediately. The third solution was developed to predict arrhythmic and non-arrhythmic disorders, so the standard 12-lead ECG is the basis for this task. Several cardiac disorders involve spatial structures and the 12-lead standard ECG is the best noninvasive approach for their analysis.

The three proposed solutions are viable in low-income countries and therefore can be extended to countries with better economic standards. Electronic designs are based on commercial components that are available in the international electronic market; this facilitates manufacturing and after-sales service, guaranteeing the sustainability of the systems.

The two solutions based on portable devices are easy to use for the subjects that require their use. Today, there is a great disposition of most human beings to use portable technology because of the impact of mobile telephony that is part of our lives. The proposed portable devices were designed to minimize their size in order to avoid discomfort and their operation requires minimal user intervention. The third solution proposes the approach of the standard resting ECG to the community to assess the trend of different parameters strongly associated with dangerous cardiac disorders. In this case, the electrocardiographic test is the traditional 12-lead ECG, so its acceptance by the subjects studied is a fact.

The three proposed solutions offer health services that do not exist or are very difficult to implement traditional methods of care for patients suffering from heart disease. It is typical for a subject suffering from cardiac arrhythmias to visit the cardiologist periodically, for instance, it could be every 3 months, but it is impossible to know what happens between two visits while the solution proposed by the authors allows to evaluate the cardiovascular system changes day by day. The second solution proposes a way to keep people with high cardiac risk due to stress or suffering from some cardiac disorder under cardiovascular surveillance. This is also very difficult to achieve in low-income countries, although in developed countries there are more compact solutions than the one proposed, although they are also more expensive.

6. Conclusions

The solutions described in this chapter are examples of simple systems to provide effective tools for cardiac disease analysis and monitoring. The approaches discussed are feasible for other chronic diseases, such as diabetes, arterial blood pressure disturbances, and respiratory diseases. The common element is the measuring of the main parameter characterizing the analyzed disease with a medical device easy to use at home. This element combined with the use of public data networks is the basis for this kind of solution.

The greatest effort has always been aimed at achieving, at a minimum cost, solutions that meet the highest current safety and quality standards.

The proposed systems have been developed and tested under real conditions without any exceptional resources. A public data network of a poor country was the support for all tests and the results were satisfactory.

Acknowledgements

The authors would like to acknowledge the collaboration of colleagues from hospitals and technical testing laboratories who supported the development of the proposed systems. Without them, it would have been impossible to get these results. The financial support of the Ministry of Science of the Republic of Cuba for the execution of the projects associated with the presented systems is also appreciated.

Conflict of interest

The authors guarantee that there is no conflict of interest with the information published in this document.

Author details

Rene Ivan Gonzalez-Fernandez[1*], Margarita Mulet-Cartaya[2], Gisela Montes de Oca-Colina[2], Jorge Aguilera-Perez[2], Juan Dayron Lopez-Cardona[3] and Jose Luis Hernandez-Caceres[1]

1 Cuban Center for Neurosciences, Havana, Cuba

2 COMBIOMED Medical Technology, Havana, Cuba

3 Universidad Carlos III, Spain

*Address all correspondence to: rigf58@yahoo.com

References

[1] Mendis S, Lindholm LH, Mancia G, et al. World Health Organization (WHO) and International Society of Hypertension (ISH) risk prediction charts: Assessment of cardiovascular risk for prevention and control of cardiovascular disease in low and middle-income countries. Journal of Hypertension. 2007;**25**:1578-1582

[2] The WHO CVD Risk Chart Working Group. World Health Organization cardiovascular disease risk charts: Revised models to estimate risk in 21 global regions. The Lancet Global Health. 2019;7:e1332-e1345. DOI: 10.1016/S2214-109X (19)30318-3

[3] Tison GH, Zhang J, Delling FN, Deo RC. Automated and interpretable patient ECG profiles for disease detection, tracking, and discovery. Circulation. Cardiovascular Quality and Outcomes. 2019, 2019;**12**:e005289. DOI: 10.1161/CIRCOUTCOMES.118.005289

[4] Macfarlane PW, Kennedy J. Automated ECG interpretation – A brief history from high expectations to deepest networks. Heart. 2021;**2**:433-448. DOI: 10.3390/hearts2040034

[5] Moraes E, Barros LP, Rodrigues AE, Pagliara AT, Carvalho AC. Pre hospital electrocardiography: Prevalence of clinically important ECG findings of a public health system in a developing country. In: 2nd International Conference on Global Tele Health. 26–28 November, 2012. Australian Tele Health Society. Sydney; 2012

[6] Abraham WT, Stevenson LW, Bourge RC, Lindenfeld JA, Bauman JG, Adamson PB, et al. Sustained efficacy of pulmonary artery pressure to guide adjustment of chronic heart failure therapy: Complete follow-up results from the CHAMPION randomized trial. Lancet. 2016;**387**(10017):453-461. DOI: 10.1016/S0140-6736(15)00723-0. Epub 2015 Nov 9

[7] Frederix I, Solmi F, Piepoli MF, Dendale P. Cardiac telerehabilitation: A novel cost-efficient care delivery strategy that can induce long-term health benefits. European Journal of Preventive Cardiology. 2017 Nov;**24**(16):1708-1717. DOI: 10.1177/2047487317732274. Epub 2017 Sep 19

[8] Ligtenberg A, Kunt M. A robust-digital QRS-detection algorithm for arrhythmia monitoring. Computers and Biomedical Research. 1983;**16**(3):273-286. ISSN 0010-4809. DOI: 10.1016/0010-4809(83)90027-7

[9] Gonzalez-Fernandez R et al. Combining ECG and pulse oximetry for newborn cardiovascular screening. Acta Scientific Medical Sciences. 2020;**4**(6):49-54

[10] Gonzalez-Fernandez R, Mulet-Cartaya M, Lopez-Cardona JD, Lopez-Rodriguez L. A mobile application for cardiac rhythm study. Computing in Cardiology Conference. 2015;**2015**:393-396. DOI: 10.1109/CIC.2015.7408669

[11] Kwok CS, Darlington D, Mayer J, Panchal G, Walker V, Zachariah D, et al. A review of the wide range of indications and uses of implantable loop recorders: A review of the literature. Heart. 2022;**3**:45-53. DOI: 10.3390/hearts3020007

[12] Lai E. Converting analog to digital signals and vice versa. In: Practical Digital Signal Processing. Newnes; 2003. pp. 14-49. ISBN 9780750657983. DOI: 10.1016/B978-075065798-3/50002-3

[13] Beyramienanlou H, Lotfivand N. An efficient Teager energy operator-based automated QRS complex detection. Journal of Healthcare Engineering. 2018; **2018**:8360475. DOI: 10.1155/2018/ 8360475

[14] Banerjee A, Shanthi Mendis V. Heart Failure: The Need For Global Health Pe rspective. Current Cardiology Reviews. 2013 May;**9**(2):97-98. Published online 2013 May. DOI: 10.2174/ 1573403X11309020001

[15] Hamm W et al. Risk prediction in post-infarction patients with moderately reduced left ventricular ejection fraction by combined assessment of the sympathetic and vagal cardiac autonomic nervous system. International Journal of Cardiology. 2017;**249**:1-5

[16] Xiaojuan X, Björn W, David GS, Galen SW, Jciech Z, Arthur JM. Jean-Philippe Couderc, Automatic QRS. Selvester scoring system in patients with left bundle branch block. EP Europace. Feb 2016;**18**(2):308-314. DOI: 10.1093/ europace/euv040

Section 2

The Far-Reaching Telehealth and Telemedicine on Pharmacy, Rehabilitation and Surgery

Chapter 4

Stakeholders of the Online Pharmaceutical Market

András Fittler, Márton Fittler and Róbert György Vida

Abstract

During the past two decades, the pharmacy supply chain has developed a new segment besides traditional "brick and mortar" pharmacies. The expansion of the internet, consumer experience in online purchases, the ease of mail order trade, and distance selling have facilitated the growth of the internet pharmacy landscape. Changes in health-seeking behavior, patient empowerment, and openness to self-diagnosis and self-treatment have also contributed to the phenomenon and were further facilitated by the pandemic. Various types of online medicinal product sellers have been published previously, however, authors have classified online pharmacies mainly according to legality and patient safety considerations. As online pharmacies show great diversity, no distinct categories can be specified, rather pharmacies on the web can be categorized by multiple aspects. Admittedly, consumer preferences, regulatory environment, and legitimacy of operation are key influencing factors. In this chapter, key aspects of categorization and nomenclature are discussed to profile different vendors on the internet.

Keywords: internet pharmacies, illegal online pharmacies, drug supply chain, patient safety

1. Introduction

Internet today is not only a resource for health information but a real opportunity to obtain medical services and pharmaceuticals due to changes in health-seeking behavior, patient empowerment, and openness to self-diagnosis and self-treatment. During the past decades, the internet has become an accepted means to procure various products, especially during the pandemic, and the pharmacy supply chain has developed a new segment beside traditional brick-and-mortar pharmacies. The main motivation lurking behind internet procurement of medications is convenience, the potential to save money, and assure client privacy. The pandemic has caused changes regarding the demand and access to medications and has facilitated self-care and self-medication behaviors among the public worldwide. Likely the experience in online purchases, the ease of mail-order trade, and distance selling has further facilitated the growing market of online pharmacies. Recent reports and a representative sample of Hungarian outpatients suggest the use of internet pharmacies and the number of individuals obtaining medications and various health products online is increasing [1], international literature data indicate the prevalence of buying prescription drugs online in the population ranges from 1 to 32% [2]. Admittedly, the COVID-19 pandemic has impacted consumer behavior and changed consumer preferences, further integrating pharmacy e-commerce in healthcare delivery [3].

Internet pharmacy is an umbrella term, while online pharmacy, e-pharmacy, e-commerce pharmacy, or cyber pharmacy often being used as synonyms. Although there is no internationally accepted definition, internet pharmacies are entities that offer and dispense nonprescription and prescription medicines direct to patients and offer products and services through an internet website [3, 4]. Distant selling of medicinal products by mail-order pharmacies has existed in the United States for more than a century [5] and during the past decades, it has extended its services online, becoming online retail mail-order pharmacies. The first legitimate internet pharmacy started its operation in 1999, however, during the past two decades rapid proliferation has been observed with the penetration of e-commerce, digital service offerings, and direct-to-consumer healthcare [3, 6].

Due to the intangible nature of the internet, the actual size of the online pharmacy market is yet relatively unknown. Thousands of internet pharmacies are accessible on the web; and as the internet is an immeasurable and low-controlled environment, a vast number of illegitimate vendors overwhelm the market of online pharmaceuticals [7, 8]. It is difficult and nearly impossible to determine the total number of active internet pharmacies, the volume of medicines sold or the actual public health impact [9], as data is not aggregated, and insights are difficult to derive from this channel [10]. This is mainly because the illegal market segment is an uncontrolled environment, with practically no restrictions regarding vendors, consumers, or products. Nearly anyone can purchase any type of medication without a prescription, medical supervision, or appropriate diagnosis, consequently compromising patient and medication safety. Hence, the globalization regarding e-commerce has enabled the creation of a "digital pharmaceutical gray market" separate and far beyond the legitimate supply chain [6]. In addition to the benefits perceived by patients, several patient safety risks are linked to the procurement of medicines outside the traditional supply chain, including questionable sourcing, poor product quality, improper storage, and transportation [11], while cybercrime including consumer fraud and data privacy issues can be noted as potential nonhealth-related risks [12]. Illegitimate online pharmacy

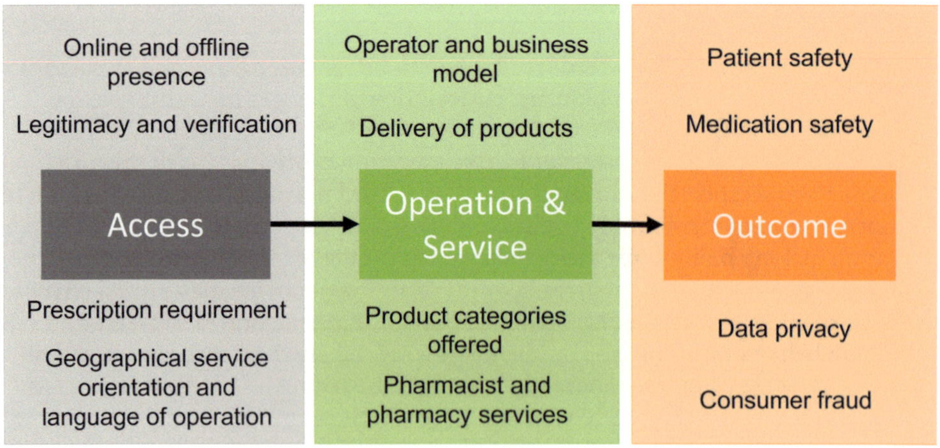

Figure 1.
Elements of evaluating internet pharmacy websites.

websites are considered the major source of substandard and falsified medications in developed countries [6, 13, 14]. Illegal actors have been using the internet as a channel of distribution and the problem of online prescription drug sales has been escalating since the mid-1990s [15]. Although, probably, it would be better to reserve the term "internet pharmacy" only for licensed legitimate websites providing legitimate professional pharmacy services, in our current chapter for simplicity, we will refer to online vendors of medicinal products as internet pharmacies.

Cyberspace is global and not local, websites can be viewed globally, and e-commerce crosses jurisdictional boundaries, consequently, internet pharmacies and purchasing of medications via the internet make regulation and governance problematic [16]. In the case of trans-border trade, the country of operation determines the licensing regulations and the quality assurance standards. Concurrently, delivery must be performed in accordance with the destination country's regulations on distance sale of pharmaceuticals. As many, likely illegal, websites are reluctant to reveal their real-world location, consumers cannot bear the responsibility of illegitimate purchases as they cannot be sure of the regulatory framework under which the website is operating [17].

Due to the lack of internationally standardized regulations the control and law enforcement of medications moving across the border is an issue, often making national authorities powerless outside their own borders. Safety issues related to online pharmacies originate from a lack of regulation. According to the FIP global survey on online pharmacy operations and distribution of medicines, more than half (n = 37, 51%) of the responding countries indicated that they had no regulations for online pharmacies, while nearly all in Africa and South-East Asia were lacking laws regulating online pharmacy operations [3].

Despite the national legal differences, there are a few internationally accepted norms. These include that prescription-only medicines cannot be dispensed without a valid physician order, and that pharmacies shall adhere to the regulations on the distant sale of medications in the destination country. Further, controlled substances (narcotics, psychotropics) and unauthorized medicines or ones not approved for sale by the national drug authority cannot be distributed, meanwhile, the sale of substandard and falsified medicines is considered a crime.

As internet pharmacy websites show great diversity, online medicine vendors can be categorized by multiple aspects. In the above, simplified process scheme, the most influential aspects of internet pharmacies are illustrated. The method of how consumers contact vendors and online availability, further regulatory framework regarding the distant sale of medicinal products are important elements of accessibility of internet pharmacy websites. The degree of interaction with customers and patients impacts the services provided by operators of the website. Finally, treatment outcome and patient safety are the primary outcome parameters of internet pharmacies (see **Figure 1**).

2. Categorization aspects of internet pharmacies and online vendors of medicinal product

2.1 Legitimacy and verification

Although sometimes used synonymously, the distinction between legal-illegal and legitimate-illegitimate online sales and purchases of pharmaceuticals must be discussed. Legitimate internet pharmacies are *registered* and possess a pharmacy license to dispense medications, further these websites are monitored and adhere to national regulations. These websites comply with the regulations of the country of operation and the country of destination where the products are shipped [7]. Websites adhering to their national jurisdictions may trade medications transborder to consumers in countries with different domestic laws. It may occur that in the destination country where a consumer is located, the online pharmacy is not registered and/or the medication is not legally sold. In these circumstances, the consumer is engaged in unauthorized or illegitimate online purchase. Even though the selling prescription drugs without valid prescription violates regulations consumers may not be aware they are obtaining drugs illegally [16]. According to LegitScript's data on a global scale, approximately 5% of online pharmacies operate in full compliance with applicable jurisdictions [18].

Illegal/rogue online pharmacies intentionally fail to comply with national or international standards and regulations. The most common and noticeable indicator of these online vendors is the sale of prescription-only medication without a valid prescription, not to say controlled (addictive) prescription drugs. These websites account for approximately 92% of all online vendors, and operators do not have legally required pharmacy licenses and sell unapproved and unregulated medications [18].

Verification is of key importance, however, may not necessarily correlate with patient- and/or medication safety issues. Unfortunately, in a relatively large proportion (n = 21, 38%) of the countries participating in a global survey, there is no established method to verify the authenticity of online pharmacies [3]. At once, verification systems are not mutually recognized internationally. The main issue related to verification systems is that they require consumer awareness, without consumer knowledge of the dangers of illegal medicines sales and the existence of verification systems, their impact on protecting patients is relatively low. Additionally, nonprofessional and unofficial verification systems may exist and the seals used to differentiate legitimate websites from illegal ones can be faked.

However, there are numerous web-based verification/accreditation/certification systems worldwide. Unfortunately, verification systems are generally not accepted internationally. Further, parallel to national and international systems approved or maintained by drug authorities, private agencies also certify that drug-selling websites and nonreputable verification services may also exist. These services differ in certification standard, coverage, business model, and certification outcome [19]. Website seals or logos provided by certificate agencies, commercially available verification services, and top-level domain names are currently available solutions for providing reliable information for consumers regarding the legal status of an online pharmacy. These methods rely on and require consumer awareness and participation at the point-of-sale [8].

Accredited or legitimate vendors display website seals as images and links acquired from national or regional agencies or authorities. The National Association of Boards of Pharmacy (NABP) initiated the Verified Internet Pharmacy Practice Site (VIPPS) program in 1999, the program is voluntary and requires payment verification. This rigorous inspection program expects mainly US-based online pharmacies to comply with relevant regulations, right to privacy, authenticate and secure prescription orders, adhere to quality assurance policy, and provide meaningful consultation with pharmacists. The majority of accredited websites (currently less than 100) in the NABP's database are open to all customers, including chain pharmacies and pure online pharmacies. The remaining are membership-only sites that belong to pharmacy benefit managers. The NABP reviews fraudulent operators and publishes a not recommended sites list as well. A European regulation applicable to the legal sale of medications via the internet was implemented in the Falsified Medicines Directive 2011/62/EU (FMD) and all EU states follow the model described by the regulation. Since 2015 internet pharmacies in the EU must be registered by national authorities and display the common recognizable security logo [16]. Additional European voluntary registers of online medicine retailers officially authorized for the mail order trade were available before the FMD for example the DIMDI logo in Germany or the Registered Pharmacy in the UK. The common EU online seal verification requires visitors to click on the image, the logo takes the visitors to registers on the authority's website where the retailers' details are displayed.

LegitScript.com is the commercial leader private company for website verification services partnering with search engines, e-commerce platforms, payment companies, and regulatory agencies. In addition to internet pharmacies, telemedicine providers, and other healthcare merchants can get certified in the healthcare merchant certification program. The website permits free public searches for consumers to check online pharmacy legitimacy. PharmacyChecker is a verification agency established in 2003, requiring voluntary application and certification fees for Canadian and international online pharmacies. The website allows price comparison among verified members that meet the standards and guidelines for pharmacy accreditation. However, a complete list of searchable database of approved members or unapproved illegal sites is not available on the company's website. It has been published that the private agency has less stringent requirements and has certified suspect online drug sellers previously [20].

The ".pharmacy" generic top-level domain was launched by NABP in the USA as an ultimate identification for safe, legal, and ethical internet pharmacy websites. As the highest level of the internet namespace, it is a built-in verification tool for credible and safe websites, and as opposed to verification/certification logos, there is no possibility to fake the pharmacy extension. Evidently, the benefits are limited if consumers are not aware of this top-level domain while navigating in the online space [8].

2.2 Online and offline presence

The click-and-brick pharmacies offer online and offline services, these websites are the virtual representation of an individual pharmacy store, chain, or grouping, for example, Boots in the UK or CVS in the USA. Meanwhile, internet-only internet pharmacies do not have a physical store that patients can enter thus websites are not linked to brick-and-mortar pharmacies. Such pure-play online pharmacies include DocMorris in Germany. Regardless of the type of operation, it is a mandatory requirement for a legitimate online pharmacy to have a physical address and the contact information must be clearly presented on the websites.

2.3 Prescription requirement

Prescription-only pharmacies request valid prescriptions, including e-prescriptions, faxed or scanned versions, written by independent medical doctor to be submitted. There are two forms of online health status evaluation methods. Prescribing/online consultation pharmacies require individuals to consult with health professionals (physician or pharmacist) employed by or affiliated to the online pharmacy to obtain prescription drugs. Some internet pharmacy websites supply medications following the completion of an online questionnaire; however, this method appears to give consumers a false sense of health assurance than providing an actual health status assessment. Although online patient questionnaires can identify certain contraindications or prevent medication errors, these instruments can be bypassed by consumers, filled with inappropriate data, or include pre-selected answers [2]. No-records online pharmacies dispense prescription drugs without any prior documentation necessary [9]. Electronic prescriptions, implemented in the jurisdictions of many countries according to a recent FIP survey [3] will further facilitate the growth of the legitimate online market.

2.4 Operator and business model

Stakeholders of the pharmaceutical e-commerce market can be further classified according to the operator of the website. Legitimate internet pharmacies (e-pharmacies) are directly linked to and operated by a licensed pharmacy business. Depending on national regulations the operator may be a local independent community pharmacy, a pharmacy/drugstore chain, or a mail-order pharmacy (USA) extending its service online. Central pharmacy portals are operated by a trade association, distributor, or franchise partner involving independent pharmacies that offer orders online and collect in-local store service.

Affiliate and aggregator websites are often listed in search engine results and can be considered dominant players in promotion of medicinal and consumer health products. These sites are operated by individuals or companies and do not deal with products listed on their websites, rather than only market another company's products by diverting customers to the merchant's site for an agreed commission fee. Aggregator websites provide the opportunity to compare products from multiple merchants and direct users to the selected page. Websites engaged in an affiliate internet pharmacy program act as influencers and receive a commission for sending traffic and sales to online merchant websites. Interestingly, only a minority of the websites in the illegal internet marketplace operate independently as 97% of rogue websites are part of an affiliate network or other grouping indicating common control [18].

2.5 Product categories offered

Distant selling of medicinal products may be limited to consumer healthcare products including nonprescription or over-the-counter (OTC) medicines, dietary supplements, and patient- and personal-care products. By default, legitimate online pharmacies offer these products without medical prescription in several countries (e.g., Hungary and Russia) [21]. However, online sale of nonprescription medications is not allowed in 19% of countries participating in a survey published by the FIP in 2021 [3]. Subject to national regulations remote retail trade of prescription-only (Rx) medicines is also available from verified internet pharmacies in numerous countries (e.g., China, Germany, India, Lithuania, USA, Sweden) [10]. Although restrictions apply to selling certain Rx pharmaceuticals remotely, such as controlled drugs (narcotics, psychotropic medicines). The development and acceptance of online sales of medicines are illustrated by the fact that high-cost specialty medicines requiring special handling and/or clinical assessment are also supplied by online outlets linked to brick-and-mortar pharmacies in most regions of the world [3].

Due to complicated global differences in medicine regulations, nonprescription medications can be further classified as pharmacist-only medicines sold by licensed outlets and requiring consultation with a pharmacist, and general sales list medicines also available from nonpharmacy outlets [16]. The majority of countries limit the supply of pharmacist-only medicines if the website is linked to a brick-and-mortar pharmacy [3]. Accordingly, the majority of the internet pharmacies can be categorized as nonprescription-only e-pharmacies or extended product portfolio OTC + Rx e-pharmacy websites. Additional stakeholders selling consumer healthcare products with no direct connection to licensed pharmacies are present on the internet. These nonpharmacy webshops include general outlets (e.g., supermarkets) and parapharmacies (e.g., druggists) offering healthcare products including nutrients, herbal products, patient- and personal-care goods. Although in some countries consumers can purchase non-prescription medicines from non-pharmacy retailers, in most instances no authorized or licensed medicines are offered by operators not holding a pharmacy license.

Some online medicinal product vendors may not sell a vast range of products and brands, but rather specialize in a single specific brand or therapeutic area. Such dedicated websites may deal only with vitamins, lifestyle and embarrassment drugs (erectile dysfunction, hair loss, obesity, etc.), dental or veterinary products, controlled drugs (e.g., alprazolam, oxycodone), and steroids.

2.6 Delivery of products

Online pharmacies may offer in-pharmacy pick-up or cooperate with nonpharmacy pick-up points (e.g., retail druggist chains). For distance sales, the logistical function can be provided by mail or courier delivery. Delivery time and cost are important aspects of online purchases and distant sales of medicinal products. In general, purchasing medications from internet pharmacies can be lengthy as the delivery may require several days or even weeks depending on the county of origin. Additional implicit or explicit expenses should be considered, as shipping costs can have a significant impact on the total expenses for low-cost item purchases. Further, in the case of transborder trade, customs fees or taxes may also apply.

2.7 Geographical service orientation and language of operation

Pharmacies can provide their services to the local community to domestic customers within a country, or trans-border to reach international markets. Websites focusing on domestic customers are monolingual, while others serving international markets can be multilingual. Legitimate internet pharmacies typically offer their services and target their sales in the national and regional jurisdiction where they are licensed [18]. Disclosure of the website operator's geographical location and contact information is an essential element of transparency and legitimacy. However, such information may be biased as several studies have demonstrated the declared physical location may not correspond to the area of domain registration [9].

Numerous websites modify the language of operation based on the geolocation of the visitor or enable international visitors to select the language of operation. As illegal online vendors are willing to ship to locations where they are not licensed and/or where they are not allowed to sell prescription drugs, multilingualism and global market orientation may be linked to illegal activity.

2.8 Pharmacist and pharmacy services

Although in most countries pharmacists are not able to access shared patient health records [3], as the level of access (e.g., medication history, laboratory results) and rights (reading or writing) increase the complexity of pharmacy services offered offline and online will further develop. The minimum "service" available on websites is basic information about the product offered, including instructions, composition, price, etc.

3. Issues related to illegitimate online vendors

The risks to humankind require a global approach and international multidisciplinary cooperation. Most importantly, (a) national regulatory frameworks are heterogeneous regarding the distance sale and online marketing of medicines, (b) national authorities are typically powerless beyond their continental borders, (c) the effectiveness of public campaigns is limited, and (d) uninformed consumers are unlikely to be able to differentiate legitimate websites from illegitimate perpetrators. Consequently, illegitimate operators provide fraudulent online services and disregard safe pharmacy standards without legal or commercial consequences worldwide [6, 9].

A comprehensive risk assessment and test purchase methodology have been developed and published by our research group culminating in a decade of robust research (Vida et al., 2020). Our findings usher beneficial, descriptive evidence regarding issues related to the uncontrolled online market, including (a) unsubstantiated health claims lacking scientific evidence and missing warnings on contraindicated conditions and drug-interactions, (b) wide availability and easy access to biological and oncological medications, and (c) quality issues due to unprofessional distribution and handling [11, 22, 23]. Several review articles (Mackey and Nayyar, 2016; Nayyar et al., 2019) support that uncontrolled perils associated with the illicit online pharmaceutical market are persistent and current legislation and law enforcement actions seemly are ineffective to battle the complex globalized illicit online pharmaceutical market. In particular, vendors of the illegal internet market utilize abusive "underground" marketing techniques including e-mail spam, manipulation of search engine results, and development of large affiliate networks [18, 24, 25].

In the case of counterfeiting and online marketing, the traditional quality assurance measures supporting medications in the legal supply chain (e.g., audits and analytical measurements), leave gaps between the manufacturing and the product use, as it is not possible to assess the quality of a drug sold online until purchased. Furthermore, normal consumers (patients) do not own laboratory instruments and professional knowledge to determine the safety and efficacy of a specific medication. Product quality issues are likely recognized later as the unwanted effects occur or the lack of desired pharmaceutical effects becomes obvious [26].

Patient safety harm associated with counterfeit or illegal medicine use can be categorized based on the quality issue and content of the products. These products may contain toxic doses of a component (e.g., glibenclamide, metformin) or a dangerous component (e.g., diethylene glycol and/or chromium) and can result in poisoning. Additionally, the poor quality of these medicines may compromise the treatment of chronic and infectious diseases (e.g., β-lactam antibiotics), causing disease progression and drug resistance. Falsified medicines may also carry microbes from other geographical locations in the world and lead to unexpected infectious diseases [14, 26].

In consideration of the manufacturing and distribution of drugs becoming more complex, modern technology-based solutions are needed to protect patients. Emerging technologies focusing on supply chain elements are under development (e.g., radio frequency identification, blockchain technologies, and edible noncloneable functions) or being implemented during the past years (e.g., serialization and the Falsified Medicines Directive in Europe and mobile-based verification of products in developing countries) [8]. However, as described in our recent research paper their efficacy outside the legitimate supply chains, such as the illegal online pharmacy market, is questionable even in developed countries [27]. Numerous publications emphasize the interdiction of internet sales of falsified and substandard medicine requires strategies yet to be developed [28]. It must be noted that several attempts to regulate the online pharmacy market (website verification databases, online logos, top generic domain name) have been introduced during the past decade, both in the USA and throughout the EU, but with limited effect upon the globalized illicit e-market of pharmaceuticals [29, 30].

Accordingly, due to the limitations of previously applied or generally used methodologies, novel approaches and methods are necessary and further research is required to develop standardized protocols to address the intrusion techniques, the prevalence, health consequences, and economic burden of substandard and falsified medicines distributed via the internet [28]. Developing technologies, such as the use of machine learning and competitive intelligence tools for market research, show a great promise in detecting and preventing the sale and distribution of substandard and falsified medicines, especially via online platforms [6].

4. Multistakeholder approach in the online pharmaceutical market

Stakeholders who can contribute to the integrity of the supply chain include organizations representing health professionals, patients and consumers, manufacturers, distributors, authorities, prevention and enforcement services (police, customs, justice), media and governments, and medicines providers (community and hospitals pharmacies). Further, search engine providers have a decisive role in evaluating and moderating search engine result pages, for example, by excluding unfair online marketing practices of illegitimate vendor sites [31]. All parties would benefit from a safe and regulated internet pharmacy market segment. Consumers and patients could take advantage of the benefits of e-commerce without evident dangers associated with illegal sellers and dubious products sold online. Pharmaceutical supply chain participants would also benefit from a safe internet pharmacy market, as infiltrated supply chains, illegal manufacturers, and distributors displace sales from legitimate pharmaceutical companies and retailers. In addition to loss of revenue, illegal and counterfeit products damage the reputation of brands, firms, and in general the perception of safety and efficacy attributed to medicines. An uncontrolled environment impacts governments and healthcare systems by diverting resources from limited health budgets due to direct and indirect health costs associated with patient harm, regulatory and enforcement actions, and patients' loss of confidence in healthcare systems.

As we aim to envision the online pharmaceutical market as a safer place for consumers and patients, multiple stakeholders should be kept in mind. This chapter gives an opportunity to the readers to familiarize themselves with the complexity of the online market segment of the pharmaceutical supply chain, a continuously developing segment with significant potential threats to healthcare systems and individuals as well. The multistakeholder aspect and various participants and services utilized by the legal and illicit actors give an uneven, rugged nature to this market that seems to be difficult to control. Admittedly, we have described and evaluated the characteristics of the surface web, however, one should not forget the additional threat associated with the uncontrolled and illegal sale of medicinal products on the deep and dark web. In this ecosystem transnational organized crime syndicates use legal services like Internet Service Providers (e.g., search engines, social media platforms, payment procedures, transportation services, and domain name registries), highlighted by the 2016 review from Mackey and Liang [6].

Seemingly, there's no golden bullet or ultimate measure that will solve the international issues related to uncontrolled online medicine sales. National regulatory approaches can decrease patient safety risks by providing an opportunity for the legal sector to grow and fighting against illegal actors. Although there are multistakeholder approaches and initiatives like Operation Pangea including law enforcement, pharmaceutical and wholesales industries, internet service sector, credit card companies, health regulators, and customs agencies; however, their regular and continuous operation would be required to increase the efficacy of their actions. Active participation of healthcare workers, including pharmacists, general practitioners, nurses, and the patients' organizations is required in this field, as the point of care interventions can easily and efficiently increase consumer awareness [7, 32, 33].

5. Conclusions

Internet pharmacies are trending in most countries and have become popular participants in the pharmaceutical supply chain, especially for consumer healthcare products. The global market size is estimated to be more than US$50 billion and is growing at an impressive rate [10]. Depending on national regulations majority of legitimate and verified websites offer non-prescription, herbal products, dietary supplements, cosmetics, etc., meanwhile, in some countries, prescription-only medicines are also available via distant selling. Unfortunately, benefits are hindered by patient safety concerns due to illegal vendors overwhelming the online pharmacy landscape.

Preferably, internet pharmacy websites should adhere to regulations set by the country of operation and the country where the products are shipped to. Internationally harmonized legal frameworks and a global internet pharmacy verification system would facilitate quality assurance and law enforcement of the transborder trade of pharmaceutical products. Physical location and contact information of the seller must be clearly stated on the website, and consultation with a licensed healthcare professional should be available for customers. If the regulatory environment permits, online vendors must require a valid medical prescription from a licensed prescriber for prescription-only medicines. Similarly, to offline interactions between the patient and the pharmacists, online vendors shall evaluate the health status of consumers prior to purchase. Website content must contain all essential information (indication and effects, dosage, contraindications, storage, etc.) required for the safe use of the products.

Although the internet pharmacy landscape is constantly developing, a better understanding of online vendors and e-pharmacy shoppers is required to maximize benefits and limit potential harms associated with online medicinal product purchases.

Funding

The research has been supported by the ÚNKP-21-5-PTE-1349, ÚNKP-21-2-I-PTE-1259, ÚNKP-21-4-PTE-1118, and ÚNKP-22-5-PTE-1730 New National Excellence Programs of The Ministry for Innovation and Technology from the source of the National Research, Development and Innovation Fund, further supported by the János Bolyai Research Scholarship of the Hungarian Academy of Sciences (BO/00238/20/5).

Conflict of interest

The authors declare no conflict of interest.

Notes and other declarations

None.

Author details

András Fittler*, Márton Fittler and Róbert György Vida
Faculty of Pharmacy, Department of Pharmaceutics, University of Pécs, Hungary

*Address all correspondence to: fittler.andras@pte.hu

References

[1] Fittler A, Vida RG, Káplár M, Botz L. Consumers turning to the internet pharmacy market: Cross-sectional study on the frequency and attitudes of hungarian patients purchasing medications online. Journal of Medical Internet Research. 2018;**20**(8):e11115

[2] Long CS, Kumaran H, Goh KW, Bakrin FS, Ming LC, Rehman IU, et al. Online pharmacies selling prescription drugs: Systematic review. Pharmacy. 2022;**10**(2):42

[3] International Pharmaceutical Federation. Online Pharmacy Operations and Distribution of Medicines. The Hague: The Netherlands, 2021

[4] Orizio G, Schulz P, Domenighini S, Caimi L, Rosati C, Rubinelli S, et al. Cyberdrugs: A cross-sectional study of online pharmacies characteristics. The European Journal of Public Health. 2009;**19**(4):375-377

[5] Khandelwal N, Duncan I, Rubinstein E, Ahmed T, Pegus C. Community pharmacy and mail order cost and utilization for 90-day maintenance medication prescriptions. Journal of Managed Care Pharmacy. 2012;**18**(3):247-255

[6] Mackey TK, Nayyar G. Digital danger: A review of the global public health, patient safety and cybersecurity threats posed by illicit online pharmacies. British Medical Bulletin. 2016;**118**(1):110-126

[7] Fittler A, Bosze G, Botz L. Evaluating aspects of online medication safety in long-term follow-up of 136 internet pharmacies: Illegal rogue online pharmacies flourish and are long-lived. Journal of Medical Internet Research. 2013;**15**(9):e199

[8] Mackey TK, Nayyar G. A review of existing and emerging digital technologies to combat the global trade in fake medicines. Expert Opinion on Drug Safety. 2017;**16**(5):587-602

[9] Orizio G, Merla A, Schulz PJ, Gelatti U. Quality of online pharmacies and websites selling prescription drugs: A systematic review. Journal of Medical Internet Research. 2011;**13**(3):e74

[10] IQVIA Consumer Health. e-Pharmacy and the New Consumer Whitepaper. 2020 https://www.iqvia.com/library/white-papers/e-pharmacy-and-the-new-consumer-whitepaper

[11] Fittler A, Vida RG, Rádics V, Botz L. A challenge for healthcare but just another opportunity for illegitimate online sellers: Dubious market of shortage oncology drugs. PLoS One. 2018;**13**(8):e0203185

[12] Miller R, Wafula F, Onoka CA, Saligram P, Musiega A, Ogira D, et al. When technology precedes regulation: The challenges and opportunities of e-pharmacy in low-income and middle-income countries. BMJ Global Health. 2021;**6**(5):e005405

[13] Gaudiano MC, Manna L, Bartolomei M, Rodomonte AL, Bertocchi P, Antoniella E, et al. Health risks related to illegal and on-line sale of drugs and food supplements: Results of a survey on marketed products in Italy from 2011 to 2013. Annali dell'Istituto Superiore di Sanità. 2016;**52**(1):128-132

[14] Blackstone EA, Fuhr JP, Pociask S. The health and economic effects of counterfeit drugs. Am Health Drug Benefits. 2014;**7**(4):216-224

[15] Inciardi JA, Surratt HL, Cicero TJ, Rosenblum A, Ahwah C, Bailey JE, et al. Prescription drugs purchased through the internet: Who are the end users? Drug and Alcohol Dependence. 2010;**110**(1-2):21-29

[16] Sugiura L. Respectable Deviance and Purchasing Medicine Online. Cham: Springer International Publishing; 2018

[17] Alwon BM, Solomon G, Hussain F, Wright DJ. A detailed analysis of online pharmacy characteristics to inform safe usage by patients. International Journal of Clinical Pharmacy. 2015;**37**(1):148-158

[18] The Center for Safe Internet Pharmacies. The Internet Pharmacy Market in 2016: Trends, Challenges and Opportunities [Internet]. He Center for Safe Internet Pharmacies (CSIP). 2016 [cited 2022 Mar 30]. Available from: https://safemedsonline.org/wp-content/uploads/2016/01/The-Internet-Pharmacy-Market-in-2016.pdf

[19] Bate R, Jin GZ, Mathur A. In whom we trust: The role of certification agencies in online drug markets. B E Journal of Economic Analysis & Policy 2014;**14**(1):111-150

[20] Liang BA, MacKey T. Searching for safety: Addressing search engine, website, and provider accountability for illicit online drug sales. American Journal of Law & Medicine. 2009;**35**(1):125-184

[21] Lobuteva L, Lobuteva A, Zakharova O, Kartashova O, Kocheva N. The modern Russian pharmaceutical market: Consumer attitudes towards distance retailing of medicines. BMC Health Services Research. 2022;**22**(1):582

[22] Vida RG, Fittler A, Mikulka I, Ábrahám E, Sándor V, Kilár F, et al. Availability and quality of illegitimate somatropin products obtained from the internet. International Journal of Clinical Pharmacy. 2017;**39**(1):78-87

[23] Vida RG, Fittler A, Somogyi-Végh A, Poór M. Dietary quercetin supplements: Assessment of online product informations and quantitation of quercetin in the products by high-performance liquid chromatography. Phytotherapy Research. 2019;**33**(7):1912-1920

[24] McCoy D, Pitsillidis A, Jordan G, Weaver N, Kreibich C, Krebs B, et al. PharmaLeaks: Understanding the business of online pharmaceutical affiliate programs. In: Proceedings of the 21st USENIX Security Symposium. 2012. pp. 1-16

[25] Leontiadis N, Moore T, Christin N. A nearly four-year longitudinal study of search-engine poisoning. In: Proceedings of the 2014 ACM SIGSAC Conference on Computer and Communications Security. New York, NY, USA: ACM; 2014. pp. 930-941

[26] Rahman MS, Yoshida N, Tsuboi H, Tomizu N, Endo J, Miyu O, et al. The health consequences of falsified medicines-a study of the published literature. Tropical Medicine and International Health. 2018;**23**(12):1294-1303

[27] Vajda P, Richter K, Bodrogi Z, Vida RG, Botz L, Kovács S, et al. Survey of workflow and cost implications of decommissioning regarding the falsified medicines directive in Hungarian hospital pharmacies. BMJ Open. 2021;**11**(11):e047193

[28] Nayyar GML, Breman JG, Mackey TK, Clark JP, Hajjou M, Littrell M, et al. Falsified and substandard drugs: Stopping the pandemic. The American Journal of Tropical Medicine and Hygiene. 2019;**100**(5):1058-1065

[29] Fadlallah R, El-Jardali F, Annan F, Azzam H, Akl EA. Strategies and systems-level interventions to combat or prevent drug counterfeiting: A systematic review of evidence beyond effectiveness. Pharmaceutical Medicine. 2016;**30**(5):263-276

[30] Hamilton WL, Doyle C, Halliwell-Ewen M, Lambert G. Public health interventions to protect against falsified medicines: A systematic review of international, national and local policies. Health Policy and Planning. 2016;**31**(10):1448-1466

[31] Fittler A, Paczolai P, Ashraf AR, Pourhashemi A, Iványi P. Prevalence of poisoned google search results of erectile dysfunction medications redirecting to illegal internet pharmacies: Data analysis Study. Journal of Medical Internet Research. 2022;**24**(11):e38957. DOI: 10.2196/38957. PMID: 36346655

[32] Fittler A, Bosze G, Botz L. Attitude of patients and customers regarding online drug purchase - a Hungarian community pharmacy survey. Orvosi Hetilap. 2010;**151**(48):1983-1990

[33] Fittler A, Lankó E, Brachmann B, Botz L. Behaviour analysis of patients who purchase medicines on the internet: Can hospital pharmacists facilitate online medication safety? European Journal of Hospital Pharmacy. 2013;**20**(1):8-12

Chapter 5

Telerehabilitation in Low- and Middle-income Countries

Intan Sabrina Mohamad and Irma Ruslina Defi

Abstract

Telemedicine is the delivery of healthcare services using information and communication technologies (ICT) to its users. Mobile communications in telemedicine or Mobile health (mHealth) is the most commonly accepted mode of telemedicine in low- and middle-income countries (LMICs) due to its affordability and user-friendly features. Telemedicine may be used to treat, prevent and monitor health conditions; as well as to promote health and educate clients. Access to medical and rehabilitation services in LMICs may be limited due to the lack of expertise, geographical locations, and sociocultural issues. Telerehabilitation (TR) may be a practical solution to circumvent these barriers in LMICs. TR providers must possess the necessary knowledge, skills, and expertise to deliver quality TR services to clients while ensuring patient safety and adhering to medical ethics and regulations. Policymakers and administrators should ensure vulnerable groups are included when making policies on healthcare services. Changes must be made to existing policies on telemedicine, in order to include all stakeholders in TR and overcome human, organizational, and technical challenges in LMICs.

Keywords: telerehabilitation, telemedicine, low- and middle-income countries, LMIC

1. Introduction

Telemedicine, also known as telehealth, eHealth, telepractice, online medicine, virtual consultation [1], or distant medicine [2] is the delivery of healthcare services using information and communication technologies (ICT) to its users. The use of mobile communications is called Mobile health (mHealth), which is the most commonly accepted mode of telemedicine in low- and middle-income (LMIC) [3, 4]. In 2020, upper-middle income countries (UMIC) like Malaysia had 40.69 million mobile subscriptions and 27 million (83.1%) internet users [4].

Telemedicine may be used to treat, prevent and monitor health conditions, as well as to promote health and educate clients [5]. Although the list is not exhaustive, applications of telemedicine have expanded beyond teleconsultations to telerehabilitation, telesurgery, telerobotics, telereferrals, telepharmacy, teletherapy, telediagnostics (telepathology, teleradiology); teleassessments, telemonitoring, telementoring, teleeducation, and telecounseling [6, 7].

Telemedicine provides faster access and communication between healthcare providers (HCPs) and patients [8, 9]. The COVID-19 pandemic has accelerated the uptake of telemedicine as it avoids direct exposure to infections, reduces traveling

 IntechOpen

time and cost [8–10], and reduces time away from work or caregiving. Sub-acute cases requiring rehabilitation and monitoring can no longer be managed in acute or rehabilitation hospitals due to competing health priorities and shortened length of stay (LOS). Telerehabilitation (TR) may be a key innovation to ensure continuity of care post-hospital discharge and reduce the global burden of disability [11–13].

The scope of TR services depends on 4Ps namely the patient, provider, policymaker, and payer. The needs of its people and healthcare system will steer the direction of telemedicine in LMIC [13]. The success or failure of TR will depend on the dynamic relationships between human, organizational, and technical factors [10, 11]. Vulnerable groups such as people with disabilities (PWDs) and the elderly in LMIC face additional challenges in accessing TR.

Sociocultural issues such as unemployment, homelessness, overcrowding, language barrier, cultural and religious beliefs; and literacy will influence the delivery and uptake of TR. Literacy does not only mean the basic ability to read and write, but also the ability to navigate ICT and contextualize information obtained from healthcare professionals (HCPs) and the media. Non-English speakers may face additional literacy disparity, as 63.2% of the information on the internet is in English [14]. TR services should be available in foreign languages so as not to exclude a significant proportion of people who are only proficient in their native language [13]. Policymakers and HCPs must ensure vulnerable groups are included when making policies on healthcare services. Existing policies and guidelines on telemedicine in LMIC are mostly physician-centric [15–17] and do not have clear policies on fee structure, insurance coverage, and financial incentives for allied health professionals (AHPs) [17]. Changes must be made to existing policies on telemedicine, in order to include all stakeholders in TR and overcome human, organizational and technical challenges in LMIC.

2. Telerehabilitation in low- and middle-income countries

2.1 Telerehabilitation requirements

TR services depend on the needs of its people and healthcare systems and are differentiated by their ecosystem and convenience. Low cost and technology, easy-to-use features, and quick responses are key to the adoption of TR in LMIC. **Figure 1**

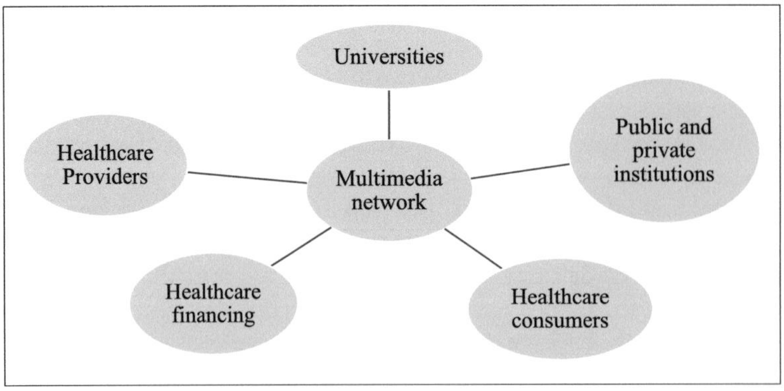

Figure 1.
Hub-and-spoke model on telerehabilitation stakeholders. (Source: Adapted from Malaysian Telemedicine Flagship Application, 2013; page 12) [7].

shows a Hub-and-spoke model and illustrates the inter-relationships among TR stakeholders.

TR requirements can be categorized into:

- Providers
- Clients
- Information and communication technologies (ICT)
- Training
- Policies and guidelines
- Outcome measures

2.1.1 Telerehabilitation providers

Although the list is not exhaustive, TR providers may include:

- Healthcare Professionals (HCPs)

  Treat patients, instead of going to health centers, these services can be accessed through ICT they give consultation, examine patients and devise a treatment plan which includes prescribing medications, therapies, and rehabilitation equipment for patients. HCP also requests laboratory tests.

- Policymakers

  Write regulations for health care providers to protect patient's rights and safety,

- Organizations, hospitals, or health centers

  Look into the runnings of TR

- Laboratories

  Process patient's samples for health care providers to access, but this can also be accessed by the patients themselves without the health care providers.

- Pharmacies

  Dispense medicine prescribed by HCPs

- Researchers

  Conduct research and studies of evidence-based practice and review policies

- Data analyzer

  Analyze data, from all of the above, such as policies, laboratories, and the information stored and transmitted in the TR process

- Hardware or software developers

  Develop technology to be used in the TR process

- Telecommunication and internet providers

  Provide connectivity between TR providers and the clients

- Artificial intelligence (AI)

The three major components of TR are clinicians, IT, and TR services. A clinical provider's role is to deliver TR services [18]. They may either be physicians, AHPs [17] such as nurses, therapists, counselors, social workers, dietitians, pharmacists or traditional and complementary practitioners, or even caregivers [11]. TR providers may be stationed at hospitals, clinics, health centers, homes [5], or online.

There should be good leadership in TR. TR providers are regarded as leaders or brand ambassadors in telemedicine; promoting and building relationships among stakeholders such as HCPs, policymakers, and hardware or software developers [18]. TR providers need to embrace new technologies such as AI (Chatbot or robots) to meet clients' exponential demand for an immediate and constant response beyond office hours. The high cost and lack of human resources to deliver TR may be substituted with pre-programmed Chatbot responses, and prerecorded audio or text messaging systems.

2.2 Telerehabilitation clients

Telerehabilitation clients may include:

- Patients

- General public

- Paid caregivers

- Family members

- Healthcare providers

PWDs and those with chronic diseases in LMIC often undergo a vicious cycle of disability, unemployment, and poverty. Family members usually become informal caregivers, since paid caregivers are costly and not sustainable. Caregivers in LMIC often have to work several jobs to support PWD in the family or give up their jobs to be full-time caregivers. Family-based rehabilitation (FBR) and community-based rehabilitation (CBR) may be realistic models of care in LMIC [11, 12]. TR facilitates FBR and CBR by empowering caregivers and HCPs in the community.

Not all PWDs can be TR clients. Patients with acute emergencies, with severe communicative disorders and no access to ICT, may need additional considerations and in-person assistance [11, 19]. TR providers must adhere to the Code of Ethics and have a duty of care to ensure patient safety prior to selecting patients as TR clients [1, 10] (see case history 1).

DOI: http://dx.doi.org/10.5772/intechopen.107449

2.3 Case history 1

Mrs. Y is an elderly lady who lives with her elderly husband, *Mr. Y* who has hearing impairment, in a village with no internet access. She has sudden left knee pain and cannot travel to the hospital on her own. *Mr. Y* informed *Nurse LN* to assess *Mrs. Y*. *Nurse LN* made a diagnosis of acute septic arthritis and called for an ambulance to transfer *Mrs. Y* to the local hospital. *Dr. HQ* (TR provider) discharged *Mrs. Y* a week later with a home exercise program, to be supervised by *Nurse LN*. *Nurse LN* (TR client) visited *Mrs. Y* weekly and taught *Mr.* and *Mrs Y* the prescribed exercises. Two months later, *Miss SN* (TR client) sent pictures and videos of *Mrs. Y* cooking and walking to *Dr. HQ* and the rehabilitation team at the hospital (TR providers) via WhatsApp.

2.3.1 Information and communication technologies

ICT is a major component of TR as it links TR providers to its users (**Figure 1**). ICT may be broadly classified into:

- Technology
- Equipment
- Combination of both (hybrid)

Information can be transmitted through the following methods:

- Synchronous
- Asynchronous
- Hybrid

2.3.1.1 Synchronous telerehabilitation

Synchronous communication is also known as sync, real-time, face-to-face (F2F) or live interaction between TR provide and its users. Synchronous TR provides immediate responses and exchange of information between two or more parties. Body language, tone of voice and better rapport can be established via live video. Illiterate and visually impaired TR clients can interact with TR providers without having to read written information, as in asynchronous TR. Any doubts, misunderstanding, and feedback can be obtained immediately via verbal communication.

Fast internet speed, adequate data capacity, and technical expertise are required in order to provide synchronous TR. The minimum broadband speed for satisfactory synchronous teleconsultation or teleeducation in Vietnam (LMIC) is 2 Mbps, whereas diagnostic images such as those transmitted in teleradiology would require a minimum of 4 Mbps2. Upper middle-income countries (UMIC) such as Malaysia, have an average download speed of wireless broadband of 15.6 Mbps to 27.6 Mbps20; which is slow compared with the average fixed internet connection speed worldwide (78.0 Mbps).

A survey conducted in 2020 revealed internet users in Malaysia used smartphones (96%), laptops/notebook/netbook (41%), and tablets (18%) for Chat Apps (97%), social networking Apps (70%), and entertainment or video Apps (55%) [4]. Some examples of apps which can be downloaded for free and have synchronous features are WhatsApp, Facebook live, FB messenger, Instagram, WeChat, GoogleMeet, Zoom, and Skype. Video conferencing and live chats can also be conducted on Chatbots and telephone. ICT user habits and trend may project how synchronous TR can be delivered in LMIC and UMIC [4, 23–25].

2.3.1.2 Asynchronous telerehabilitation

Asynchronous communication is also known as async or store-and-forward communication [7]. Information can be exchanged between two or more parties without the involvement of live or immediate responses. Asynchronous information can be stored and edited beforehand and viewed later. There is no time-pressure and it does not require everyone to be present at the same time. Caregivers in LMIC often have to juggle between work commitments and providing care for PWDs. Asynchronous TR may be more acceptable to caregivers and patients who cannot commit to appointment scheduled within office hours or when there are ICT limitations for synchronous TR. Clients who are introverts, shy or not well-versed in F2F communication may also find asynchronous TR more appealing.

Some examples of asynchronous communication are SMS, email, and voice or video recordings. Prerecorded lectures, webinars, and YouTube videos are popular modes of asynchronous information, which can be useful in LMIC.

2.3.1.3 Hybrid telerehabilitation

At times, TR clients may require a hybrid of synchronous and asynchronous telerehabilitation in order to fulfil their needs. Most smartphones contain apps with hybrid features, such as WhatsApp, Facebook live, FB messenger, Instagram, WeChat, Google Meet, Zoom, and Skype [4]. These apps are popular in LMIC as they can be downloaded for free, easy to use, and can be accessed on multiple ICT devices such as smartphones, desktops, laptops, and tablets.

2.3.1.4 Mobile health

Mobile health (mHealth) is the most commonly accepted telemedicine method among patients with chronic diseases in LMIC [3], because of its affordability and easy access in rural and poor communities [2, 8–13, 20, 21, 27]. Systematic reviews on mHealth interventions in rehabilitation [23, 24] showed positive outcomes in the following domains:

- Exercise training
- Gait training
- Self-management systems
- Measurement tools

TR clients can receive reminders via SMS, access information and services; monitor biochemical markers, physiological readings, and behaviors from their mobile phones [23, 24]. The most commonly used mobile phone Apps in LMIC are Facebook, WhatsApp, Viber, Skype, Zoom, and GoogleMeet [4, 22–25], mainly due to its free and user-friendly features.

Some examples of free mHealth Apps in South East Asia are MySejahtera, MorChana, Vietnam Health Declaration, PeduliLindungi, and StaySafe PH26. These apps are used to monitor public health, disseminate information and provide health education to the public. Mobile Apps such as Doc2us and Halodoc from Malaysia and Indonesia respectively, provide teleconsultation, teleprescription, and medication delivery to its user at an affordable fee. Such telemedicine services are not only timely during the COVID-19 pandemic but also help reduce the workload on government-funded health centers [26].

A critical factor that must be considered in LMIC is data affordability. In Malaysia, a prepaid mobile phone plan of 2.5 Gb data costs RM 26 (USD 6.22) per month, while a postpaid Plan with unlimited data costs RM68 (USD 16.28) per month [27]. The main difference between a Pre-paid and a postpaid mobile plan is the payment schedule. The former only provides mobile service based on the load of the purchase (pay-as-you-use), while the latter is billed at the end of the monthly subscription and is based on data consumption. Prepaid plans are more affordable for users in the lower economic group (B40) such as in Malaysia, a country where the minimum wage is RM 1200 per month or USD 9.57 per day. Similar observations have been reported in other LMIC [11–13, 25, 28, 37–44].

2.3.1.5 Assistive technology

Assistive technology (AT) is any item, place of equipment, software program, or product system that may be used in rehabilitation to increase, maintain, or improve the functional capabilities of persons with disabilities (PWDs) [23, 24]. AT features may be built into smartphones such as switch and voice controls for PWDs with limited limb and verbal functions. Other accessibility features include magnifying or bolding fonts and texts for visually impaired people.

Some wearable devices have AT features that use wireless or Bluetooth technologies. PWDs with limited limb functions such as tetraplegics or amputees may use a wearable device such as the *GlassOuse* and *Bite Switch* (mouse) to connect and operate their mobile phones, computers, tablets, and smart television using Bluetooth technology [29] (**Figure 2**). TR providers in LMIC require training and funding for AT to be useful in their practice.

2.3.1.6 Robotic technologies

Although robotic technologies may be useful in rehabilitation, their affordability makes them neither feasible nor sustainable in low-resource settings. Evidence-based reviews comparing robotic technologies with standard care interventions did not show long-term significant differences in locomotor training for walking after spinal cord injury and stroke or upper limb function after stroke [30]. TR providers in LMIC may have to consider other affordable alternatives to robotic technologies.

2.3.2 Training

Delivering TR services requires specific competencies, which may not necessarily be taught to HCPs in their profession [11]. In addition, there is a big shortage of AHPs

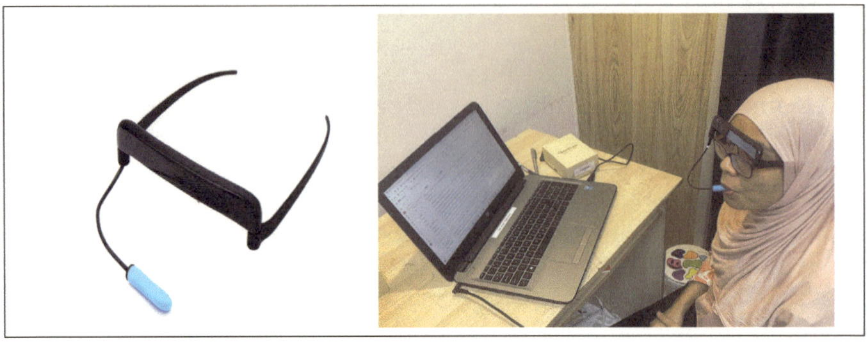

Figure 2.
GlassOuse *is worn like a pair of glasses and connects to mobile phones, computers, tablets, and smart TVs via Bluetooth. The user moves her head from side to side to navigate the cursor on the screen and bites on the* Bite Switch *(in cyan) to click items on the computer similar to a computer mouse. (*Photo by Intan Sabrina*).*

such as physiotherapists (PTs), occupational therapists (OTs), speech and language pathologists (SLPs) and audiologists in LMIC, especially in rural areas [11, 12]. There should be a TR coordinator for every TR activity in order for TR program(s) to succeed and be sustainable.

Guidelines on telepractice by AHPs are few [5, 11, 17, 30]. For example, only 10–20% of SLPs tend to use telepractice in India and only 3% of SLPs in Croatia had completed formal training related to telepractice in SLP services [11]. Organizations in LMIC should provide training and credentialing procedures for TR providers on a regular basis to suit the evolving needs of TR clients [31]. The IFNR Task Force (2021) cautioned that not everyone with a smartphone can deliver teleneurorehabilitation (TNR). They also noted that standardizing functional assessments through teleassessments may prove to be a challenge.

Training in TR can be divided into three main groups:

- HCPs
- Patients/caregivers
- IT support/technical assistant

HCPs must be trained to obtain informed consent from patients and caregivers and how to document TR activities [6]. Telemedicine service is voluntary and should allow clients to opt out at any point of the telemedicine service. Patients and caregivers in LMIC and rural areas usually require guidance, training, and on-site assistance before TR services can be delivered. The level of assistance should be determined beforehand, such as the need for interpreting language(s) or dialects, setting up ICT devices such as keeping their mobile phones charged [28] and ensuring clients have adequate mobile data and network coverage. TR clients in LMIC need to be briefed on the prerequisites of a conducive telemedicine environment [19, 28, 32]. Ideally, the latter should be a quiet room or corner, with minimal distractions from other family members and good network coverage. Any fees and costs involved in the TR service must be declared at the outset by the TR provider.

IT support and infrastructure are critical components of TR service(s), but may be limited in LMIC. Quick solutions such as on-the-job (OTJ) training among HCPs or appointing IT representatives in each unit or department may be useful to bridge gaps in IT support. HCPs who are not trained in ICT may have to switch roles from becoming TR providers to TR clients. ICT training and technology-transfer in TR may be conducted via teleeducation and telementoring.

2.3.3 Policies and guidelines

Since the COVID-19 pandemic, many countries around the world have updated their policies on telemedicine. Telemedicine guidelines should not be physician-centric and must cater for the needs of AHP, patients, and their caregivers. These guidelines must cover points of service such as healthcare settings, homes, or community-based worksites [5].

A scoping review of telemedicine guidelines in South East Asia (SEA) revealed most countries had guidelines on clinical governance, confidentiality, ICT infrastructure, data security, record keeping, and licensing [6]. However, only Singapore and Indonesia have policies on telemedicine fee structure, insurance coverage, or reimbursement for medical practitioners. Policymakers and organizations should have clear billing and coding processes designated for TR so that payers can reimburse costs to TR providers [5], especially those offered by AHPs.

Most guidelines on telemedicine tend to regulate HCPs, rather than the technologies, platforms, or types of telemedicine services [1, 6, 33]. Telemedicine guidelines should have clear credentialing, privileging and regulatory requirements for licensure, certification, and use of telemedicine and its applications [5, 6, 11]. Mobile apps and internet of things (IoTs) are usually regulated by Medical Device Acts in the country they are registered (MDA) [34–36]. TR providers should adhere to their respective organizations and regulating bodies to ensure the safe and effective delivery of TR services to their clients [1, 5, 6, 15–17].

3. Setting up telerehabilitation services in low- and middle-income countries

TR providers must identify the service(s) which can be converted to TR exclusively or as a hybrid model. Clear inclusion and exclusion criteria for patient selection must be outlined in the TR Standard Operating Procedure (SOP) [5, 32, 33]. A feasibility study should be conducted to familiarise every stakeholder prior to the roll-out of the TR service [19]. Any hiccups should be addressed accordingly.

There are four main phases in telerehabilitation [32, 33]:

- Precontact (Pre-C)
- Actual contact (AC)
- Postcontact (Post-C)
- Data collection

Pre-C activities comprise calling the TR client and introducing the purpose of TR, obtaining verbal and/or written consent, clarifying contact details of the TR client and determining the medical or rehabilitation requirements. Details on the date, time, platform of AC and fee should also be conveyed clearly to the TR clients during the Pre-C phase. Technical assistance (TA) such as ICT literacy, translation, or physical assistance should also be pre-determined in the Pre-C phase. TA may comprise any family member, neighbor or the local HCPs closest to the TR client's home.

Pre-C activities may be simplified by using questionnaires or assessment tools, which may be sent via email, text message and/or Google Doc formats. For example, in a tele home visit, TR clients can send measurements, pictures and videos of their home environment to their Occupational Therapist (OT) via email or WhatsApp messages or videos. The OT can then make the necessary recommendations for home modifications, prescribe rehabilitation equipment and arrange for a F2F assessment if required. Another example is when TR clients send audio recordings of their vocal exercises to their Speech Therapist or Audiologist prior to AC sessions.

A standard script, template, and checklist [32] would be useful to standardize communication between both parties. All communications and interventions involving TR clients should be documented clearly in the client's medical records [5, 6, 19, 25, 32, 33].

AC activities may range from teleconsultation to teleassessment, teletherapy, telemonitoring and teleeducation. Details such as patient identification, diagnoses, medications, investigation results, progress report, rehabilitation equipment, funding options and treatment needs should be addressed in the AC phase and documented in the clients' medical records. TR providers should determine the outcome measures, assessment tools and equipment involved in the AC activities. Several trials of Pre-C and AC activities should be conducted prior to the roll-out of TR services to address pitfalls and additional TR requirements.

Post-C activities may include documenting and storing data collected in the Pre-C and AC phases, referrals to other parties, teleprescriptions of medications, information and/or home-based programs to TR clients, issuing medical certificates, and other activities similar to F2F consultations. All TR activities must be documented clearly and securely stored to ensure patient confidentiality, data security, and storage.

Finally, TR providers must be trained in data collection on TR activities and compare them with those in the standard-care pathway(s). The TR coordinator should review all TR services periodically and provide feedback to all stakeholders for quality assurance (QA) and improvements [32].

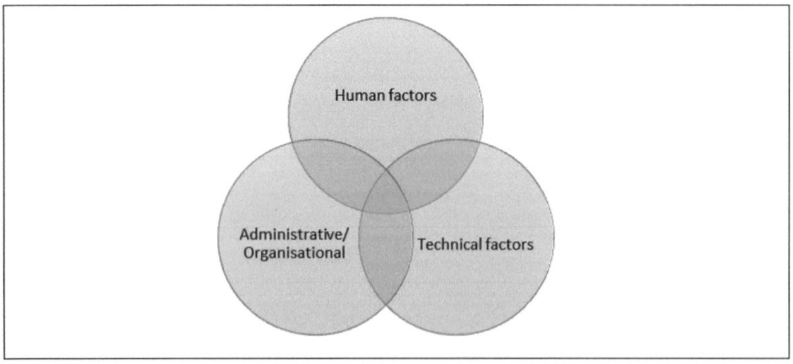

Figure 3.
Challenges in telerehabilitation in low- and middle-income countries (Source: Adapted from Leochico et al. 2020. Telerehabilitation Challenges in Developing Country; ***Table*** *2, page 10 [12]; and IFNR Research Task Force et al. 2021. TeleNeurorehabilitation During COVID-19 in LMICs, 2021;* ***Table*** *2, page 4 [11]).*

Challenges	Malaysia5,18 (UMIC)	Indonesia19,20,40–43 (LMIC)	Philippines13 (LMIC)	India10 (LMIC)	Africa23,36–39 (LIC)
Human/personal factors					
• Lack of knowledge/awareness in TR	Yes	Yes	Yes	Yes	Yes
• Lack in ICT skills/literacy	Yes	Yes	Yes	Yes	Yes
• Poor participation	Yes	Yes	Yes	Yes	Yes
• Poor adherence	Yes	Yes	Yes	Yes	Yes
• Resistance to change	Yes	Yes	Yes	Yes	Yes
• Lack of satisfaction	Yes	Yes	Yes	Yes	Yes
• Lack of trust/effectiveness/quality	Yes	Yes	Yes	-	Yes
• Paper/physical culture	Yes	Yes	Yes	Yes	Yes
• Concerns on ICT/ethics/medicolegal	Yes	Yes	Yes	-	Yes
• Lack of TR leadership	Yes	Yes	Yes	-	Yes
Organizational/administrative factors					
• Lack of guidelines/ law	No	No	Yes	Yes	Yes
• Lack of governance	Yes	Yes	Yes	-	Yes
• Lack of financing/reimbursement	Yes	Yes	Yes	Yes	Yes
• Lack of technical support/training/literacy	Yes	Yes	Yes	Yes	Yes
• Lack of ICT resources	Yes	Yes	Yes	Yes	Yes
• Time constraints/busy schedule	Yes	Yes	Yes	Yes	Yes
• Lack of partnerships among stakeholders	Yes	Yes	Yes	-	-
Unclear roles	-	-	Yes	-	Yes
• Accountability	Yes	Yes	Yes	-	Yes
• Liabilities	-	Yes	Yes	-	Yes
• Environmental constraints/limited space	Yes	Yes			
Technical factors:					
1. **ICT-related**					
• Slow internet speed	Yes	Yes	Yes	Yes	Yes
• Limited ICT coverage in rural areas	Yes	Yes	Yes	Yes	Yes
• ICT failure/ limitations	Yes	Yes	Yes	Yes	Yes
• Dependence on electricity/battery-life/ internet	Yes	Yes	Yes	Yes	Yes
• Hardware/software limitations	Yes	Yes	Yes	Yes	Yes
• Unclear video display	Yes	Yes	Yes	Yes	Yes
• Inadequate infrastructure	Not all	Not all	Not all	Not all	Not all

• Licenced property of mobile Apps/ TR software	Yes	Yes	Yes	Yes	Yes
• High cost	Yes	Yes	Yes	Yes	Yes
• Limited AI	Yes	Yes	Yes	Yes	Yes
2. Service delivery					
• Lack of correlation with F2F assessment	Yes	Yes	Yes	Yes	Yes
• Difficulty in physical examination and treatment	Yes	Yes	Yes	Yes	Yes
• Lack of capacity for empathy	Yes	Yes	Yes	Yes	Yes
• Time-consuming	-	Yes	-	-	Yes
3. Data security					

AI – artificial intelligence; Apps – applications; F2F – face-to-face; ICT – information and communication technologies; LIC – low-income country; LMIC – lower middle-income country; TR – telerehabilitation; UMIC – upper middle-income country.
NB: This summary is based on a scoping review on Telemedicine Guidelines in South East Asia by the authors and published in Front. Neurol. 11:581649. doi: 10.3389/fneur.2020.581649

Table 1.
Challenges to deliver telerehabilitation in low-and middle-income countries.

4. Challenges to deliver telerehabilitation in low- and middle-income countries

Challenges to deliver telerehabilitation in LMIC [11, 12, 37–44] can be categorized into human, organizational, and technical factors (**Figure 3**). These factors usually overlap with one another, such as guidelines and laws on telemedicine (human and organizational); lack of digital knowledge and skills (human and technical); and lack of technical support and training (organizational, and technical). **Table 1** is a summary comparing challenges to delivering TR in five LMIC. The recurring themes in LMIC are lack of ICT training and infrastructure, lack of political will, and time-constraint. TR providers should review these challenges regularly and provide solutions so that TR services can be improved and be sustainable. A scoping review on telemedicine guidelines in South East Asia by Sabrina and Defi suggested that there should be a comprehensive and universal telemedicine guideline for any country to adopt based on the local context [6].

Challenges	Solutions
Human/personal factors Lack of knowledge/skills in ICT and TR. Lack of partnerships among stakeholders. Negative attitude towards TR. Paper/physical culture. Concerns on ICT/ethics/ medicolegal Lack of TR champion/leadership	• Train HCPs in general and specific TR services. • Simplify user experience. • Normalize the use of technology • Use familiar technology (WhatsApp video, telephone). • Use teleeducation and telementoring. • Start a small group of TR providers, then expand gradually. • Build rapport/therapeutic relationships with TR clients. • Engage with stakeholders and perform feasibility studies on TR. • Conduct cost-benefit analysis of TR and compare with existing service. • Try hybrid TR service(s) into existing system. • Devise a visual and written framework for remote musculoskeletal assessments to modify traditional tests. • Provide continuous feedback and motivation to TR clients to increase participation and discipline. • Have clear inclusion and exclusion criteria for TR. • Create local policies, guidelines, and laws on specific TR services. • Enforce clinical governance. • Provide an online helpdesk. • Appoint internal medicolegal advisors. • Appoint champions of TR for each TR service. • Have regular feedback sessions and rotations in TR leadership.
Organizational/administrative factors Lack of policies/guidelines/law Lack of governance Lack of financing/reimbursement Lack of ICT resources/technical support/training/literacy Time constraints/busy schedule Unclear roles • Accountability • Liabilities Environmental constraints/limited space	• Create local policies, guidelines, and laws on specific TR services. • Enforce clinical governance. • Lobby for TR funding with relevant authorities/governing bodies. • On-the-job ICT training for HCPs in TR services. • Have practice runs prior to starting TR service with TR providers and users. • Appoint champions of TR as ICT support staff. Try hybrid TR service(s) into existing system. Policies on TR should outline clear roles and responsibilities of TR providers with each organization/TR service. Reorganize or share working space. Review space utility and efficiency with other stakeholders/departments.

Challenges	Solutions
Technical factors:	• Policymakers and government need to invest in ICT
ICT-related	infrastructure.
Slow internet speed	• Organizations should allocate resources and IT support for TR
Limited ICT coverage in rural areas	providers and clients.
ICT failure/limitations	• ICT equipment must be maintained to ensure safety and
• Dependence on electricity/	effectiveness.
battery-life/internet	• Ensure only licenced Apps are used to avoid medicolegal
• Hardware/ software limitations	implications.
• Unclear video display	• Use free mobile apps familiar to TR clients.
• Inadequate infrastructure	• Try hybrid TR service(s) into existing system.
Licenced property	• Devise a visual and written framework for remote
• Mobile Apps	musculoskeletal assessments to modify traditional tests.
• TR Software	• Provide online measurement tools and sensors to measure force,
High cost/limited AI	position, and sound for assessments.
1. **Service delivery**	• Maintain eye-contact and provide continuous feedback and
• Lack of correlation with F2F	motivation to TR clients to build rapport.
assessment	Schedule TR service(s) into existing system.
• Difficulty in physical	• Ensure data privacy, storage, retrieval, and sharing follow federal
examination and treatment	and state laws and guidelines.
Lack of capacity for empathy	• Ensure compliance with professional organization or society.
Time-consuming	• Use authentication and/or encryption technology.
2. **Data security**	• Limit data access to privileged personnel.

Table 2.
Recommendations to overcome barriers and challenges to telerehabilitation in low- and middle-income countries.

5. Recommendations and future threats

Telerehabilitation will continue to be an integral component of health services in LMIC across the world. Digital health is the new norm. It is projected that mHealth will be a key player in complementing and adding value to healthcare services globally, particularly in LMIC [4, 10, 11, 25, 41]. Current trends in digital technologies indicate that mHealth is the go-to option in LMIC. Advances in AI, algorithms, and mobile apps may replace human-to-human interactions. Thus, HCPs should be equipped with the necessary skills to embrace the changing trends in healthcare delivery, especially those which do not require physical presence or touch.

In conclusion, TR in LMIC is challenging. However, affordable and quick solutions such as free mobile apps may overcome barriers in TR.

DOI: http://dx.doi.org/10.5772/intechopen.107449

Author details

Intan Sabrina Mohamad[1,2,3]* and Irma Ruslina Defi[4]

1 Department of Rehabilitation Medicine, Hospital Serdang, Selangor, Malaysia

2 Regen Rehab Hospital, Petaling Jaya, Selangor, Malaysia

3 Rehabilitation Medical Unit, Tung Shin Hospital, Kuala Lumpur, Malaysia

4 Department of Physical Medicine and Rehabilitation, Padjadjaran University, Bandung, Indonesia

*Address all correspondence to: drintansabrina@gmail.com

References

[1] Malaysian Medical Council Advisory on Virtual Consultation (During The Covid19 Pandemic). Available from: https://mmc.gov.my/wp-content/uploads/2020/04/MMC_virtualconsultationADVISORY.pdf

[2] Regulating the Management of Distant Medicine (Circular 49) Circular No. 49/2017/TT-BYT. Ministry of Health, Vietnam. Available from: https://hethongphapluat.com/circular-no-49-2017-tt-byt-dated-december-28-2017on-telemedicine.html

[3] Sahu M, Grover A, Joshi A. Role of mobile phone technology in health education in Asian and African countries: A systematic review. International Journal of Electronic Healthcare. 2014;7:269. DOI: 10.1504/IJEH.2014.0.64327

[4] Malaysia Digital Marketing Statistics. General Internet Statistics. 2021. Available from: https://digitalinfluence.com/malaysia-digital-marketing-statistics-2020-2021/

[5] Brennan D, Tindall L, Theodoros D, Brown J, Campbell M, Christiana D, et al. Blueprint for telerehabilitation guidelines. International Journal of Telerehabilitation. 2010;**2**(2):31-34. DOI: 10.5195/ijt.2010.6063

[6] Intan Sabrina M, Defi IR. Telemedicine guidelines in South East Asia – A scoping review. Frontiers in Neurology. 2021;**11**:581649. DOI: 10.3389/fneur.2020.581649

[7] HIMS. Blueprint – Towards excellence in health information management. In: Health Informatics Center, Planning Division, Ministry of Health. Malaysia; 2013. Available from: https://www.who.int/goe/policies/malaysia_hims_blueprint_2013_b.pdf

[8] Buabbas AJ, Albahrouh SE, Alrowayeh HN, Alshawaf H. Telerehabilitation during the COVID-19 pandemic: Patients and physical therapists' experiences. Medical Principles and Practice. 2022;**31**(2):156-164. DOI: 10.1159/000523775

[9] Wotton R, Bonnardot L. Telemedicine in low-resource settings. Frontiers in Public Health. 2015;**3**:5-6. DOI: 10.3389/fpubh.2015.00003

[10] Istepanian RSH, Woodward B, Richards CI. Advances in telemedicine using mobile communications. Engineering in Medicine and Biology Society, 2001. Proceedings of the 23rd Annual International Conference of the IEEE. Volume 4. DOI: 10.1109/IEBS.2001.1019600. Available from: https://www.researchgate.net/publication/3958008

[11] Srivastava A, Swaminathan A, Chockalingam M, Srinivasan MK, Surya N, Ray P, et al. Teleneurorehabilitation During the COVID-19 pandemic: Implications for practice in low- and middle-income countries. Frontiers in Neurology. 2021;**12**:667925. DOI: 10.3389/fneur.2021.667925

[12] Leochico CFD, Espiritu AI, Ignacio SD, Mojica JAP. Challenges to emergence of telerehabilitation in a developing country: A systematic review. Frontiers in Neurology. 2020;**11**:1007. DOI: 10.3389/fneur.2020.01007

[13] Babatunde AO, Abdulazeez AO, Adeyemo EA, Uche-Orji CI, Saliyu AA. Telemedicine in low and middle income countries: Closing or widening the health

inequalities gap? European Journal of Environment and Public Health. 2021; **5**(2):em0075. DOI: 10.21601/ejeph/1077

[14] Usage statistics of content language for websites. UNESCO Institute for Statistics. 2021. Available from: https:// w3techs.com/technologies/overview/ content_language

[15] Laws of Malaysia Act 564. Telemedicine Act. 1997. Available from: https://www.google.com/search?q=telemedicine+act+1997&rlz=1C1CHBF_enMY1000MY1000&oq=telemedicine+&aqs=chrome.1.69i57j35i39l2j0i512l4j69i61.4054j0j4&sourceid=chrome&ie=UTF-8

[16] Law of the Republic of Indonesia Number 11 of 2008 Concerning Electronic Information and Transactions. Undang-undang Republik Indonesia Nomor 11 Tahun 2008 Tentang Informasi Dan Transaksi Elektronik. 2008. Available from: https://zaico.nl/files/RUU-ITE_english.pdf

[17] Laws of Malaysia Act 774. Allied health professions Act. 2016. Available from: https://nutrition.moh.gov.my/wp-content/uploads/2019/10/Akta_AHP_Akta-774.pdf

[18] Alghatani KM. Telemedicine implementation: Barriers and recommendations. Journal of Scientific Research and Studies. 2016;**3**(7):140-145

[19] Agence d'évaluation des technologies et des modes d'intervention en santé (AETMIS). Telehealth: Clinical Guidelines and Technological Standards for Telerehabilitation. Report prepared by Gilles Pineau, Khalil Moqadem, Carole St-Hilaire, Robert Perreault, Éric Levac, and Bruno Hamel, with the collaboration of Hélène Bergeron, Alexandra Obadia and Lorraine Caron (AETMIS 06-03). Montréal: AETMIS. 2006. p. x

[20] Average download speed of broadband wireless in Malaysia in 2020, by mobile service provider. Available from: https://www.statista.com/statistics/1051857/malaysia-average-wireless-download-speed-of-internet-provider/ {Accessed: 9 March 202]

[21] Sianipar BH. Kebijakan pengembangan telemedisin di Indonesia. Kajian Kebijakan dan Hukum Kedirgantaraan. 2015:42-62. DOI: 10.30536/9786023181339.3

[22] Suksmono AB, Sastrokusumo U, Mengko. J TLR, Pramudito T, Oktowaty S. Overview of telemedicine activities in Indonesia: Progress and Constraints. Proceedings. 6th International Workshop on Enterprise Networking and Computing in Healthcare Industry – Healthcom 2004 (IEEE Cat. No.04EX842). 2004

[23] Marcolino MS, Oliveira JAQ, Novillo-Ortiz D. The impact of mHealth interventions: Systematic review of systematic reviews. 2018. DOI: 10.2196/ mhealth.8873. Available from: https:// www.ncbi.nlm.nih.gov/pmc/articles/ PMC5792697/

[24] Dicianno BE, Parmanto B, Fairman AD, Crytzer TM, Yu DX, Pramana G, et al. Perspectives on the evolution of mobile (mHealth) technologies and application to rehabilitation. 2015. DOI: 10.2522/ ptj.20130534. Available from: https:// pubmed.ncbi.nlm.nih.gov/24925075/

[25] Mar M, Morris C, Scott RE. WhatsApp guidelines – what guidelines? A literature review. Journal of Telemedicine and Telecare. 2019;**25**(9): 524-529

[26] Lee B, Ibrahim SA, Zhang T. Mobile Apps leveraged in the COVID-19 pandemic in East and South-East Asia:

Review and content analysis. JMIR mHealth and uHealth. 2021;**9**(11):e32093. DOI: 10.2196/32093. Available from: https://mhealth.jmir.org/2021/11/e32093

[27] The 5 best post-paid plan in Malaysia. Available from: https://www.trustedmalaysia.com/best-postpaid-palns-malaysia/

[28] Jack CL, Mars M. Ethical considerations of mobile phone use by patients in Kwazulu-Natal: Obstacles for mHealth? African Journal of Primary Health Care & Family Medicine. 2014; **6**(1);607-613. DOI: 10.4102/phcfm.v6i1.607

[29] GlassOuse – Head Mouse. Spectronics inclusive learning technologies, Australia. Available from: https://www.spectronics.com.au/product/glassouse-head-mouse)

[30] Engkasan JP. Cochrane evidence on rehabilitation using robotic technology [Internet]. 2019. Available from: CochraneRobotics_201https://rehabilitation.cochrane.org/sites/rehabilitation.cochrane.org/files/uploads/cochrane_robotics_2019_2.pdf9_2 [Accessed: 2022-07-05]

[31] Anil K, Freeman JA, Buckingham S, et al. Scope, context and quality of telerehabilitation guidelines for physical disabilities: A scoping review. BMJ Open. 2021;**11**:e049603. DOI: 10.1136/bmjopen-2021-049603

[32] Canadian stroke best practice recommendations telestroke implementation toolkit. 2020. Available from: https://www.heartandstroke.ca/-/media/1-stroke-best-practices/csbpr7-virtualcaretools-13may2020

[33] Garis Panduan Pelaksanaan Klinik Virtual (Virtual Clinic) di Hospital. Available from: file:///C:/users/intansabrina/downloads/garispanduan_pelaksanaan_klinik_virtual_(virtual_clinic)_di_hospital.pdf

[34] Laws of Malaysia Act 737 Medical Device Act. 2012. Available from: http://www.agc.gov.my/agcportal/uploads/files/Akta%20737%20-%20kelulusan%20TP.pdf

[35] Laws of Malaysia Act 738. Medical Device Authority Act. 2012. Available from: http://www.agc.gov.my/agcportal/index.php?r=portal2/lom&menu_id=b21XYmExVUhFOE4wempZdE1vNUVKdz09&page=15

[36] Regulatory Guidelines for Telehealth Products. Medical devices branch; health sciences authority. 2019. Available from: https://www.hsagov.sg/docs/default-source/hprg-mdb/regulatory-guidelines-for-telehealth-products-rev-2-1.pdf

[37] Hamad WB. Current position and challenges of e-health in Tanzania: A review of literature. Global Scientific Journals. 2019;7(9):364-376

[38] James O, Felix C, Ngozi I, Tonia O, Ekwueme CO, Agwuna KK. Telemedicine and biomedical care in Africa: Prospects and challenges. Nigerian Journal of Clinical Practice. 2016;**20**(1):1-5. DOI: 10.4103/1119-3077.180065

[39] Chifamba N. A scoping review on the challenges of Telemedicine implementation the Southern Africa. 2018. DOI: 10.13140/RG.2.2.32011.23842.

[40] Arthur G, Erika K-M, Nagla R, Isaac R, de Beer J. Artificial intelligence (AI) deployments in Africa: Benefits, challenges and policy dimensions. The African Journal of Information and Communication. 2020;**26**:1-28. DOI: 10.23962/10539/30361

[41] Moeloek NF, Ekatjahjana W. Permenkes No. 20 Tahun 2019 tentang Penyelenggaraan Telemedicine antar

Fasilitas Pelayanan Kesehatan. Ministry of Health. 2019. Available from: https://www.researchgate.net/publication/338428993

[42] Ariyanti S, Kautsarina K. Techno-economic study on telehealth in Indonesia. Buletin Pos dan Telekomunikasi. 2017;**15**:43-54. DOI: 10.17933/bpostel.2017.150104

[43] Bali S. Barriers to Development of telemedicine in developing countries. In: Heston TF, editor. Telehealth. London: IntechOpen; 2018. Available from: https://www.intechopen.com/chapters/64650. DOI: 10.5772/intechopen.81723

[44] Purwaamijaya BM,Wijaya A, Shadani SB. Perceptions and prospective analysis of artificial intelligence and its impact on human resources in the Indonesian industry 4.0. In: Proceedings of The 1st International Conference on Sustainable Management and Innovation, ICoSMI 2020, 14-16 September 2020, Bogor, West Java, Indonesia; 14-16 September 2020; Bogor. Belgium: EUDL; 2021

Chapter 6

Telesurgery and Robotics: Current Status and Future Perspectives

Sudhir Kumar Singh, Jyoti Sharma, Lokavarapu Manoj Joshua, Farhanul Huda, Navin Kumar and Somprakas Basu

Abstract

The concept of telehealth has revolutionized the healthcare delivery system. Based on this concept, telesurgery has emerged as a promising and feasible option, providing surgical care to remotely located patients. This has become possible by advancements in the robotic system combined with the cutting-edge technology of telecommunication. Since the ability to perform telepresence surgery was hypothesized, consistent development and research in this novel area have led to the beginning of telesurgical care, which can fulfill the demand for surgical care in remote locations. In addition to the benefits of robotic-assisted minimally invasive surgery, telesurgery eliminates geographical barriers, which helps patients have better access to quality surgical care. It may reduce the overall financial burden by eliminating the travel expense of the patients, providing expertise through the telepresence of experienced surgeons, and reducing the operating room personnel. The telesurgical approach is also being utilized for telementoring, i.e., real-time guidance and technical assistance in surgical procedures by highly skilled surgeons. Despite the numerous technological improvements in telesurgery, its widespread implementation in clinical setting still lags, mandating the identification of the offending factors that limit its clinical translation.

Keywords: telesurgery, robotic surgery, medical robotics, telemedicine, remote surgery

1. Introduction

Telehealth and telemedicine involve transferring expertise, through which patients can be examined, monitored, and treated without transporting the patient. Telemedicine is based on data acquisition, storage, transfer, processing, and display. This breakthrough came after the revolution in communication technology, such as high-speed data connections and management information systems [1, 2]. Patients can communicate with doctors from their homes using technology or a telehealth kiosk. Nowadays, telemedicine is an integral part of health services in many countries, and upcoming hospitals will attract patients from all over the world without geographical restrictions.

2. Telesurgery

The concept of telemedicine has been applied to provide surgical care to remotely located patients and is termed "Telesurgery" or "Telepresence Surgery" or "Remote Surgery" [3]. Initially considered as a "science fiction," it has now been materialized and will continue to be the reality in today's era. This revolutionized surgical care delivery has become possible by advancements in the robotic system. Since the establishment of the robotic surgery, the surgeon typically controls these robots by staying by the patient's side. In telesurgery, the robotic system still remains in direct contact with the patient, whereas the surgeon sits on a console at a remote location and performs the surgical task. As a backup, a surgical team remains in the operating room to proceed with the surgery as and when required [4]. Here, the advanced communication technology enables the surgeon to control the endoscopic camera and manipulate the robotic arm attached to the patient cart with real-time feedback. This emerging surgical system requires advanced wireless networking and robotic technology to perform the surgery [5]. The main objective of telesurgery is to eliminate unnecessary travel for patients and accompanying persons, apart from providing high-quality surgical care from expertise worldwide.

3. Evolution of telesurgery

The concept of telesurgery came into existence since U.S. National Aeronautics and Space Administration (NASA) started exploring the possibility of providing treatment to the astronauts in space long back in 1970 [6]. The invention of the endoscope, followed by the development of a video computer chip that allowed the magnification and projection of images onto television screens, was a breakthrough in introducing laparoscopic surgery [7]. This minimally invasive approach changed the era of surgery and created a possibility for evolution of telesurgery.

In the late 1980s, Scot Fisher and Joseph Rosen hypothesized the ability to perform telepresence surgery using a robotic system. Computer-assisted surgical tools have emerged after constant advancement in surgical instruments and techniques, followed by a gradual evolution from automated biopsy robots to high-end modern robotic surgical systems for visceral surgery (like the ZEUS Surgical System and the da Vinci System). The development of AESOP (automated endoscopic system for optimal positioning) followed by the ZEUS operating system from computer motion was an outstanding achievement in the development of robotic surgery. A parallel innovation of SRI green telepresence, which was refined further by Intuitive Surgical, conferred in the revolutionary development of the current da Vinci System [8]. Implementation of the telesurgery concept in a broader way could be possible after introducing mainly two robotic systems, i.e., the ZEUS Surgical System by Computer Motion and the da Vinci Surgical System by Intuitive Surgical. These modern robotic systems work on a master-slave technology where the surgeon sits at a console kept a few feet away from the patient cart, enabling the surgeon to view real-time three-dimensional imaging of the operative site. Complex software translates the surgeon's hand movement and manipulates the robotic arm accordingly, attached to the articulating surgical instruments and endoscope [9].

After merging with Computer Motion in 2003, Intuitive Surgical dominated the robotic surgical market and discontinued the Zeus platform as the da Vinci robot had several advantages over it. As in laparoscopic surgery, depth perception was a significant problem resolved substantially by the da Vinci system using a 3D immersive camera, while the Zeus system has a 2D screen display. Furthermore, the da Vinci system controls the surgical instrument using an "Endowrist," which mimics wrist

Year	Description
1920	The term "Robot" was first introduced by a Czech playwright "Karel Capek" in his hit play, "Rossum's Universal Robots."
1979	The Robot Institute of America sets a definition of the robot as "A reprogrammable, multi-functional manipulator designed to move materials, parts, tools, or specialized devices through various programmed motions for the performance of a variety of tasks."
1980	The "Green SRI telepresence surgical system" was developed by a joint venture of Stanford Research Institute (SRI) & National Aeronautics and Space Administration (NASA) Ames Research Center.
1984	Scot Fisher and Joseph Rosen were the surgical robotics pioneers who proposed the idea of using robotic arms to do telesurgery and researched in collaboration with NASA.
1985	The first industrial robot developed for clinical application was modified "PUMA 200" (Programmable Universal Manipulation Arm; Unimation, Stanford, California, USA) to precisely execute CT-guided brain biopsies.
1992	The "ROBODOC" (Integrated Surgical Systems, Sacramento, CA, USA) was developed with modification of the basic principles of the PUMA arm and was approved for hip replacement surgery.
1994	The "AESOP" (Computer Motion, Inc., Santa Barbara, CA, U.S.A.) was the first robotic surgical tool approved by the US Food and Drug Administration for laparoscopic surgery
1991-1997	"PROBOT" was developed by Harris et al. to perform transurethral prostate resection with ultrasound guidance.
1997	The prototype of "da Vinci Surgical System" was developed by Intuitive Surgical, Sunnyvale, CA.
2000	The "da Vinci Surgical System" (Intuitive Surgical, Sunnyvale, CA) was commercialized and approved for laparoscopic surgery.
2001	The "Zeus Surgical System" (Computer motion, Goleta, California, USA) was approved for laparoscopic surgery.
September 2001	The first trans-Atlantic procedure (known as "Operation Lindbergh") was Robot-assisted laparoscopic cholecystectomy using the Zeus Robotic platform. A surgeon in New York (USA) operated on a patient in Strasbourg (France).
2003	After the merger of Intuitive Surgical & Computer Motion, Zeus robotic platform was discontinued.
February 2003	The world's first telerobotic surgical service was established between St. Joseph's Healthcare Hamilton, a teaching hospital affiliated with McMaster University, and North Bay General Hospital, a community hospital 400 km away.
2006-2014	The next generation of the da Vinci surgical system i.e. "da Vinci S," "da Vinci Si," and "da Vinci Xi" were developed in years 2006, 2009, and 2014 respectively.
2017	The "Senhance" surgical system (TransEnterix, Morrisville, NC, USA) received FDA approval in October 2017 for laparoscopic abdominal procedures.
2017	NAVIO robotic system by Smith and Nephew 2020 for semi-autonomous joint arthroplasty.
2020	MAKO robotic system by Stryker was released for join arthroplasty.
2020	CorPath robotic intervention arm for use in coronary intervention during COVID pandemic

Table 1.
Historical timeline of the evolution of robotic system and telesurgery.

movement with natural movement with seven-degree freedom. The da Vinci Xi™ (Intuitive Surgical, 2014) is the most recent iteration of da Vinci systems, which has been redesigned to be more ergonomic and thinner and have well-arranged robotic arms to conserve space. Moreover, it has been upgraded with fluorescence imaging and near-infrared technology to better visualize vessels, tissue perfusion, and bile duct. Still, there is a lack of haptic feedback, which needs further improvement.

In usual robotic surgeries, where both console and robotic arms are directly connected to several meters of cable wire, there is no time lag in communication because data transmission from the console to the surgical device and back to the console is almost instantaneous. Thus, the surgeon sees his movements on the computer interface as he performs the surgery. When robotic telesurgery was conceptualized, the primary concern was the time delay in communication between the surgeon console and surgical robot due to moving the surgical system to a more remote location. Thus, the surgeon's real-time interventions could be milliseconds or even seconds behind the visualization of the operating field, which can lead to catastrophic outcomes during surgery. As proved in studies, a time lag of more than 150–200 milliseconds is harmful [10]. So seamless robotic telesurgery requires robust communication media between console and robot with negligible latency. To provide safe telesurgery services, collaborating with the telecommunications sector to build a secure, dependable, high-speed data transmission across enormous distances with unnoticeable delays is of utmost importancc.

The world's first telesurgery was the "Lindbergh Operation," a transatlantic cholecystectomy on a 68-year-old female patient in Strasbourg, France, performed on September 7, 2001 by Professor Jacques Marescaux in New York City. ZEUS system was used for this landmark surgery, and France telecom provided the spare fiber optic ATM (automated teller machine) lines to minimize the latency and optimize connectivity. The average time delay during surgery was 135 milliseconds, which is impressive considering the data traveled over 8600 miles (14,000 kilometers) from the surgeon's console to the surgical system and back [11]. This milestone in surgery was a big inspiration for establishing the first dedicated telerobotic surgical service in Canada. Since then, various robotic telesurgeries have been performed worldwide.

The timeline of evolution of the robotic system and telesurgery has been summarized in **Table 1**.

4. Benefits of telesurgery

Telesurgery is an extension of the telemedicine/telehealth concept that has become possible with the advancement of the surgical robot and sophisticated telecommunication technology. So the benefits of telesurgery encompass the inherent advantage of telehealthcare as well as robotic-assisted minimally invasive surgery, which are mentioned below:

I. Benefits related to the Minimal Invasive Approach include less amount of blood loss, shortened hospital stay, shorter recovery, and early return to work [12].

II. Benefit related to robotic-assisted minimally invasive surgery (i.e., teleoperation) includes:

a. Ergonomical posture of the surgeons with more dexterity than conventional laparoscopy.

b. Enhances the accuracy of motion as operators' physiological tremors can be filtered out in real time with accelerometer technology [13].

c. High-resolution (3-D) cameras allow surgeons to see close-ups of surgical sites that are not easily accessible [14].

d. Robotic arm provides easy access to hard-to-reach areas such as the pelvis.

e. Improved surgical accuracy reduces the chances of damage to surrounding structures and significantly reduces the risk of blood loss and infection [13, 14].

III. Specific benefits related to telesurgery include:

a. Delivery of high-quality surgery to remote settings, such as underserved rural areas, battlefields, and space stations.

b. Provides an opportunity for patients to receive surgical care by surgical experts from all over the world without going outside of their local hospitals. It is beneficial for patients for whom medical travel is not feasible due to financial constraints, travel-related health risks, travel restrictions, or time delays.

c. Real-time collaborations between surgical professionals from various healthcare facilities can benefit patients who require complicated microsurgical techniques and other complex surgeries.

d. Telesurgery may be a potential solution to the global shortage of competent surgeons.

e. During the COVID-19 era, apart from the benefit related to the need of lesser number of operating room staff in robotic surgery, the main benefit of telesurgery was the physical separation of the surgeon from the patients, thus reducing the interpersonal contact and spread of infection [15]. Telesurgery could also provide care when travel restrictions during a pandemic are the main reasons limiting medical care.

5. Limitations of telesurgery

Being a novel concept for delivering surgical care, telesurgery is still in its nascent phase and needs continuous upgrading. At present, the following factors pertinent to telesurgery are a major hindrance to the widespread use of this technology:

1. Time lag or latency: This vital issue is related to telecommunication and is mainly due to data transmission over a network and video coding and decoding. This time delay is directly proportional to the distance between two far-reaching locations. It has a propensity for surgical error and puts the patient's safety in danger.

A time lag of fewer than 100 milliseconds is considered an ideal latency time that a dedicated telecommunication system can achieve. A latency time greater than 300 milliseconds produces significant inaccuracies in instrument handling. Research suggests that a simple telesurgical procedure can be safely performed without any significant surgical inaccuracy with a time lag of up to 700 milliseconds [16].

2. Difficulty in procurement and maintenance of equipment.

3. Purchase of robotic systems is a major obstacle worldwide, mainly for third-world countries, because of inflated costs.

4. Establishing a robust global network to connect every part of the world is a big obstacle to initiate telesurgical services. Affordability of high-speed telecommunication is also a big problem, especially in developing nations.

5. Cyber security threats: Hijacking of telecom networks in telesurgery has surfaced as a major concern in the recent years that can compromise the patient's safety.

6. Various legal and ethical concerns can be raised when surgery is done without an interaction between the patient and the operating surgeon, who belong to different countries and have different regulatory bodies/acts related to medical care [17].

7. As telesurgery needs the collaboration of multiple medical organizations, billing issues will be a big problem and will require a decent agreement among them.

6. Scope of advancement in telesurgery

Innovation of robotic platforms opened up the path for clinical translation of the concept of telesurgery and went side by side with the advancement in the robotic system. Further advancement in telesurgery needs the incorporation of various emerging technologies.

6.1 Haptic feedback

Tactile feedback has been a big concern since the advent of laparoscopic surgery and continues to be the Achilles heel in Robotic surgery. Here the surgeon touches the tissue with a long instrument having a hinge that goes inside the patient's body through the ports. This series of interfaces of contact with instruments at various levels leads to degradation in the haptic feedback, which is necessary for precise and delicate tissue manipulation. This can be achieved by upgrading the technology of the human-machine interface (HMI) and sensor-based robotic instruments, reflecting the force of instruments on surgeons' hands [18]. There is ongoing research for making a perfect haptic-enabled telesurgical system. It also requires a seamless network-based communication that can send the data of hand motion and instrument-tissue contact from the surgeon to the patient and the other way around. An alternative to overcome this feedback problem is haptic-assisted training, which requires shared control of two master HMIs and one slave robot [19].

6.2 A 3-D visual feedback system

Although it appears that haptic feedback is vital in manipulating delicate tissues, today's upgraded versions of robotic systems are still inefficient in providing this tactile input appropriately. In addition, the relevance of haptic feedback in robot-assisted performances of surgical tasks is yet to be proved. It has been hypothesized that visual feedback of local tissue deformation caused by tension, retraction, or needle insertion can compensate for the lack of sensory force feedback [20]. The 3-D display system can provide this high-definition visual feedback, but further improvement is required in this aspect.

6.3 High speed and quality telecommunication

The quality of telesurgery depends on the quality of presentation of the information transmitted in the form of digitized data from one center to another. The quality of shared data and latency depends upon the bandwidth (i.e., the capacity of data flow) of the network used to relay the processed data. It can be accomplished by a telecommunication network having wide bandwidth, minor delay, slight jitter, and minimal data loss. The network-level quality of service (QoS) control is also required, ensuring bandwidth reservation for telesurgery [21]. The integration of recently available high-speed 5G internet could meet the required bandwidth and reduce the time lag issue that plagues telesurgery.

6.4 Internet of things (IoT)

Remote monitoring in the healthcare industry is now feasible owing to IoT-enabled devices, which can keep patients safe and healthy while allowing clinicians to provide superior care. As sensor technology is improving gradually, IoT devices can also be incorporated into surgical devices, which can enable the recording of intraoperative events and the movement of instruments [22]. By analyzing the data created by these devices by artificial intelligence technology, procedures can be standardized by identifying the most appropriate use of surgical devices, which will help in ensuring the safety of surgery but requires proper validation before incorporation into telesurgery.

6.5 Concept of "one-to-many" remote surgery

This concept can be perceived as an expert surgeon seated in the master control room remotely, performing surgeries on multiple patients simultaneously. It is helpful for surgeries that require a combined approach, i.e., robotic-assisted minimal invasive and an open approach during different steps of the procedure. For example, the expert sitting in master control will perform specific steps requiring robotic assistance in patient A present at one hospital and then switch to take control of another surgical robot attached to patient B at a different hospital. Meanwhile, the rest of the steps requiring an open approach for patient A will be completed by the onsite local surgical team [23]. By using this concept, further attempts can be made to plan complex surgeries, mimicking the production line of car manufacturers, by transferring the control of robotic arms in a predestined sequence to a group of surgeons sitting in their master control room far from each other and skilled in specific steps of surgery.

6.6 Artificial intelligence in telesurgery

Artificial intelligence (AI) has transformed various industries in the past decade. The incorporation of AI into telesurgery is a brand-new concept that has sparked a lot of interest as a part of the surgical procedure that can be automated. Thus, AI reduces the cognitive and physical burdens of the surgical team and can increase the efficiency of surgery by reducing the operative time and increasing accuracy [24]. Simultaneously, it can also decrease the required number of staff in the surgical team. The utilization of AI in other industries has led to a substantial increase in efficiency, but its role in surgical procedures has not yet been proven. A significant amount of adaptation and further research is required to prove its performance and build up confidence in its use in surgical care.

7. Clinical application of telesurgery

Several projects researching the feasibility and practicability of telesurgery on human patients were completed at the beginning of the twenty-first century. Because of various obstacles in the clinical utilization of telesurgery, it has not picked up its pace and is still in the developmental phase. The first dedicated telesurgery center was established in Canada, and at present, North America is leading the market in telesurgery [25]. Globally, every human being has the right to access all the recent surgical facilities present worldwide, and telesurgery is the critical innovation fulfilling these promises. But such facilities are not readily available in the developing countries and the rural parts of developed countries. It is a paradox that the secluded population worldwide that can benefit from telesurgery is also the one that cannot afford it due to high cost or lack of essential telecommunication facilities. But it is expected that in the near future, this problem will be alleviated as the internet access is rapidly expanding and various new manufacturers of affordable robotic systems are emerging.

Patients' perspective about telesurgery is pretty promising as most of them are very enthusiastic about the concept of using the robot for surgeries. This inclination toward new technology results from the projected benefits of smaller incisions with better cosmetic outcomes, shorter hospital stays, faster recovery, and fewer complications because of the precise movement of the robotic instrument during surgery. Still, this technology needs further advancement and scrutiny by noble clinical trials with a higher evidence level.

Telesurgery has opened up the opportunity of treating patients who require immediate medical attention regardless of their location. This could prove lifesaving in extreme conditions such as space and battlefields where getting a usual hospital is impossible. However, many obstacles stand in accomplishing this vision, such as installing the robotic system in such places and providing a robust connection to run the telesurgery proficiently with negligible latency. Various research studies are going on to test the feasibility and clinical implication at such extreme locations.

For astronauts on the deep-space mission, many surgical emergencies such as fatal injuries, appendicitis, intracranial hematoma, or kidney stones can occur, which mandate urgent operations then and there. So for such space missions, telesurgical assistance should be considered. But again, the signal delay will be a detrimental factor due to the vast distance between the earth and the space station. An added problem is the feasibility of robotic surgery in a zero-gravity environment. NASA is carrying out a series of missions in an undersea laboratory, Aquarius, simulating the extreme environmental condition found in space. Some substantial progress has been achieved in teleoperation, control of the surgical robot, and other challenges related to space surgery, such as the behavior of the organs and bodily fluids in zero gravity, but it's still a long road ahead of us [26].

Similarly, on the battlefield or in a natural disaster situation, telesurgery can offer a solution to provide surgical care at the site of injury and can save many lives. A semiautomated telerobotic device known as "Trauma Pod" has been created for such scenarios, which may conduct lifesaving surgeries and stabilize wounded soldiers on the battlefield. These are designed to be deployed rapidly in such unfavorable situations. These robots can also act as assistants, like a scrub nurse, in the operating room. These scrub nurse robots are automated to do different tasks such as changing tools, dispensing equipment, and tracking supplies. Various trials are going on to see the feasibility and further advancement in these trauma pods. Though these are currently being tested for first aid treatment such as putting intravenous lines, performing hemostasis, protecting airways, and placing monitor devices, we are hopeful, that the robot will be able to move beyond the current first-aid procedures [27].

8. Telementoring and telestration: a new domain for surgical training

The concept of telesurgery has opened up a new way of real-time teaching and training of surgical fellows. With this sophisticated communication technology, an expert surgeon present remotely mentors a trainee surgeon sitting in the operating room by controlling the endoscope to control the field of view throughout the entire procedure, as and when required. This unique way of training is known as "telementoring," which is considered an ideal method of skill-sharing and training [28]. An associated but slightly different method of real-time teaching is termed "telestration," in which the expert guides the trainees by freehand sketching or pointing out the structure by marking it over the trainees' video monitor. The remote surgeon and the surgeon with the patient will both have identical views of the surgical field [29]. At present, the Canadian Surgical Technologies & Advanced Robotics (CSTAR) is the leading facility globally, providing training via surgical telementoring and telestration. Some telesurgeons are also developing computer-based training modules that can be shared over the Internet.

Although robotic telesurgeries have been adopted since the beginning of the twenty-first century, telesurgery is not commonly used worldwide due to a lack of facility or proper training. So a robust training program is mandatory to make it available worldwide, which simultaneously ensures the patient's safety. It not only includes the training of the surgeon, but the whole surgical team, including nursing staff, OR technicians, anesthetists, and information technology technicians. Team training is necessary to attain the best clinical results. Even after a few successful robotic or telemanipulation surgeries, most surgeons will revert to traditional methods if they do not have qualified assistance from nurses and anesthesiologists. Comparative to conventional operations, these telesurgeries are technically demanding and need a well-trained surgical team, with each member an expert in their domain.

The training program's goal for robotic and telesurgery procedures should be focused on stepwise training of the surgeon. Like the traditional basic surgical skill program, this includes system training by didactic lectures, dry and wet laboratory training, and advanced procedure-specific training. After proficiently learning each step, the trainee should move on to the next level of surgical telemanipulation. Simultaneously, each step should undergo evaluation for the quality and clinical safety of the patient. Many training centers have developed and suggested adopting an objective-based curriculum for the training of surgical teams. Apart from providing training to young surgeons, these robotic and telesurgical training programs will promote academic writing and scientific publication.

9. Cost: benefit analysis

From a hospital-centric healthcare delivery model to a more sustainable and effective patient-centric model has been made possible with the introduction of telesurgery. It has revolutionized healthcare delivery by expanding it into a global patient base. However, cost remains a significant challenge hindering its global acceptance, especially in low and middle-income countries. The total expenses can be categorized into the initial investment and maintenance costs. Initial investment includes the cost of the robotic system, infrastructure development, and the cost of procurement of equipment and disposables.

Until now, Intuitive Surgical company's da Vinci system has been the best known and most used system. The estimated cost of a top-of-the-line robotic system ranges from $ 1 to 2.5 million. According to Intuitive Announces First Quarter Earnings, 6920 da Vinci Surgical Systems have been installed worldwide as of March 31, 2022 [30].

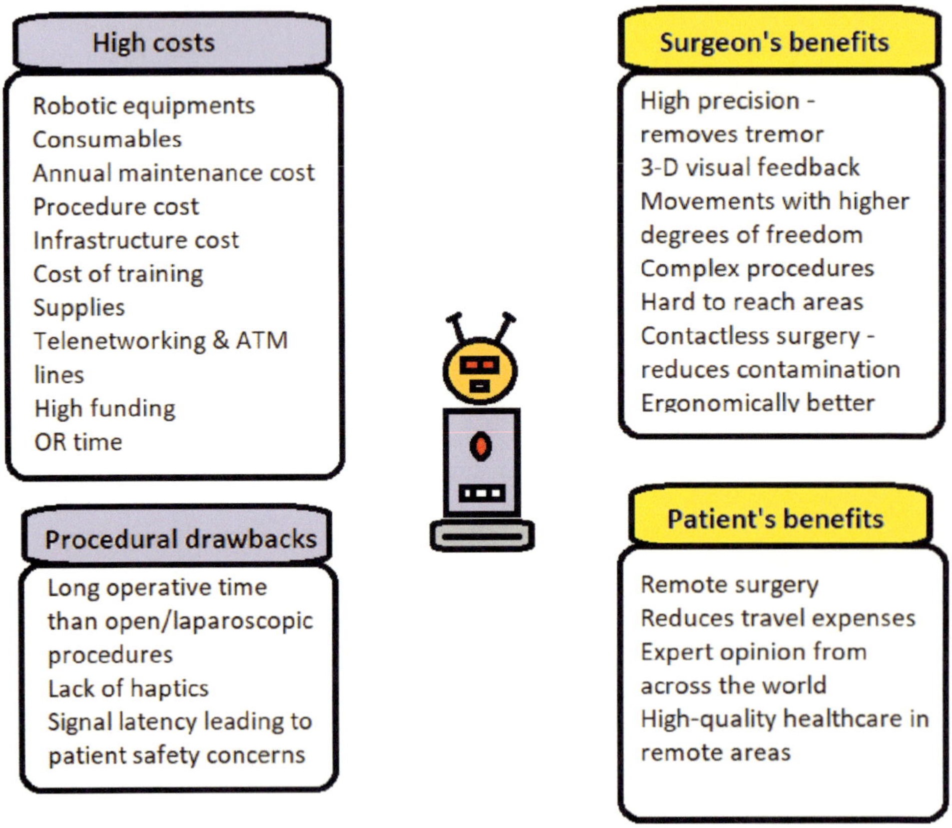

Figure 1.
Cost-benefit analysis.

The annual maintenance cost of these robotic systems is also very high. US hospitals spend $ 1000–4000 more per robot-assisted case than in endoscopic or minimal access and open procedures [31, 32]. Apart from the recently launched "Senhance" surgical system, companies such as Stryker Corporation, Hansen Medical, Verb Surgical, and Mazor Robotics are the leading companies in the robotic-assisted telesurgery market, which challenges the monopoly of Intuitive Surgical. It is believed that this competition will significantly decrease the cost of robotic systems, equipment, disposables, and maintenance in the near future.

Despite the high cost, it has been assumed that robotic surgery would be cost-effective in the long term by reducing postoperative recovery and hospital stays. Until now, most studies evaluating the cost-benefit analysis of robotic surgery are only observational studies. Concrete evidence from well-designed randomized clinical trials is needed in confirming the cost-effectiveness of robotic surgery vis-a-vis laparoscopic or open surgery.

Establishing a high-speed and quality telecommunication service is another area of high investment in telesurgery. It will be determined by the distance between the telelinked centers. In Operation Lindbergh, the estimated cost for 1-year availability of the ATM lines ranged between $100,000 and $200,000 [33]. With advancements in communication technology, its cost is also expected to decrease with time, making telesurgery and robotics available to a larger population.

Apart from the technological expenses, there is an added expense for training the surgical staff. Procedural cost, cost of additional supplies, anesthesia, and medicines required for surgery are the additional costs. It is not easy to justify these costs based only on the clinical outcome and shorter recovery time. Currently, on an objective assessment, the cost factor overwhelms the benefits associated with telesurgery. But if analyzed based on healthcare and patient outcomes, the benefits certainly outweigh the costs. The future looks promising in terms of overall cost reduction, which will make telesurgery acceptable throughout the world (**Figure 1**).

10. Conclusion

In the coming era, the goal of providing health facilities to all will be fulfilled by incorporating telemedicine and telesurgery facility into the health care system. In providing telehealthcare, setting up the facility for telesurgery requires a comparatively more robust network channel and affordable surgical robots. Apart from taking care of the scarcity of expert surgeons in remote places, it will also give freedom to choose the desired surgeon for the patient. Telesurgery may save time and money of patients and their families while improving health outcomes. Treating injured soldiers in the combat zone and astronauts in space are the added benefits of telesurgery. This technology would also allow trainee surgeons to perform surgery under the supervision of expert surgeons without jeopardizing the patient's safety. With future advancements in robotic technology, including haptic and visual feedback coupled with a 5G network, telesurgery could revolutionize health care and surgical treatment around the globe.

Acknowledgements

The authors would like to acknowledge the Department of General Surgery.

Conflict of interest

The authors report no conflict of interest.

Author details

Sudhir Kumar Singh, Jyoti Sharma, Lokavarapu Manoj Joshua, Farhanul Huda, Navin Kumar and Somprakas Basu*
All India Institute of Medical Sciences, Rishikesh, India

*Address all correspondence to: somprakas.surg@aiimsrishikesh.edu.in

References

[1] Becevic M, Sheets LR, Wallach E, McEowen A, Bass A, Mutrux ER, et al. Telehealth and telemedicine in Missouri. Missouri Medicine. 2020;**117**(3):228-234

[2] Nelson R. Telemedicine and telehealth: The potential to improve rural access to care. The American Journal of Nursing. 2017;**117**(6):17-18. DOI: 10.1097/01.NAJ.0000520244.60138.1c

[3] Bashshur R, Shannon G, Krupinski E, Grigsby J. The taxonomy of telemedicine. Telemedicine Journal and E-Health. 2011;**17**(6):484-494. DOI: 10.1089/tmj.2011.0103. Epub 2011 Jun 30

[4] Choi PJ, Oskouian RJ, Tubbs RS. Telesurgery: Past, present, and future. Cureus. 2018;**10**(5):e2716. DOI: 10.7759/cureus.2716

[5] Xia SB, Lu QS. Development status of telesurgery robotic system. Chinese Journal of Traumatology. 2021;**24**(3):144-147. DOI: 10.1016/j.cjtee.2021.03.001 Epub 2021 Mar 13

[6] Arora S, Allahbadia GN. Telesurgery: Windows of opportunity. International Journal of Health Sciences (Qassim). 2007;**1**(1):81-88

[7] Lane T. A short history of robotic surgery. Annals of the Royal College of Surgeons of England. 2018;**100**(6_sup):5-7. DOI: 10.1308/rcsann.supp1.5

[8] George EI, Brand TC, LaPorta A, Marescaux J, Satava RM. Origins of robotic surgery: From skepticism to standard of care. JSLS. 2018;**22**(4):e2018.00039. DOI: 10.4293/JSLS.2018.00039

[9] Antoniou GA, Riga CV, Mayer EK, Cheshire NJ, Bicknell CD. Clinical applications of robotic technology in vascular and endovascular surgery. Journal of Vascular Surgery. 2011;**53**(2):493-499. DOI: 10.1016/j.jvs.2010.06.154

[10] Mohan A, Wara UU, Arshad Shaikh MT, Rahman RM, Zaidi ZA. Telesurgery and robotics: An improved and efficient era. Cureus. 2021;**13**(3):e14124. DOI: 10.7759/cureus.14124

[11] Brower V. The cutting edge in surgery. Telesurgery has been shown to be feasible--now it has to be made economically viable. EMBO Reports. 2002;**3**(4):300-301. DOI: 10.1093/embo-reports/kvf083

[12] Roy S, Evans C. Overview of robotic colorectal surgery: Current and future practical developments. World Journal of Gastrointestinal Surgery. 2016;**8**(2):143-150. DOI: 10.4240/wjgs.v8.i2.143

[13] Carpenter BT, Sundaram CP. Training the next generation of surgeons in robotic surgery. Robotic Surgery: Research and Reviews. 2017;**4**:39-44. DOI: 10.2147/RSRR.S70552

[14] Palep JH. Robotic assisted minimally invasive surgery. Journal of Minimal Access Surgery. 2009;**5**(1):1-7. DOI: 10.4103/0972-9941.51313

[15] Bailo P, Gibelli F, Blandino A, Piccinini A, Ricci G, Sirignano A, et al. Telemedicine applications in the era of COVID-19: Telesurgery issues. International Journal of Environmental Research and Public Health. 2021;**19**(1):323. DOI: 10.3390/ijerph19010323

[16] Xu S, Perez M, Yang K, Perrenot C, Felblinger J, Hubert J. Determination of the latency effects on surgical

performance and the acceptable latency levels in telesurgery using the dVTrainer((R)) simulator. Surgical Endoscopy. 2014;**28**:2569-2576. DOI: 10.1007/s00464-014-3504-z

[17] Stanberry B. Telemedicine: Barriers and opportunities in the 21st century. Journal of Internal Medicine. 2000;**247**(6):615-628. DOI: 10.1046/j.1365-2796.2000.00699.x

[18] Schleer P, Kaiser P, Drobinsky S, Radermacher K. Augmentation of haptic feedback for teleoperated robotic surgery. International Journal of Computer Assisted Radiology and Surgery. 2020;**15**(3):515-529. DOI: 10.1007/s11548-020-02118-x. Epub 2020 Jan 30

[19] Butt A, K, Augestad KM. Educational value of surgical telementoring. Journal of Surgical Oncology. 2021;**124**(2):231-240. DOI: 10.1002/jso.26524

[20] Jourdes F, Valentin B, Allard J, Duriez C, Seeliger B. Visual haptic feedback fortraining of robotic suturing. Front Robot AI. 2 Feb 2022;**9**:800232. DOI: 10.3389/frobt.2022.800232

[21] Parsaei MR, Mohammadi R, Javidan R. A new adaptive traffic engineering method for telesurgery using ACO algorithm over software defined networks. European Research in Telemedicine/La Recherche Europeenne en Telemedecine. 2017;**6**(3-4):173-180

[22] Abujassar RS, Yaseen H, Al-Adwan AS. A highly effective route for real-time traffic using an IoT smart algorithm for tele-surgery using 5G networks. Journal of Sensor and Actuator Networks. 2021;**10**:30. DOI: 10.3390/jsan10020030

[23] Tian W, Fan M, Zeng C, Liu Y, He D, Zhang Q. Telerobotic spinal surgery based on 5G network: The first 12 cases. Neurospine. 2020;**17**(1):114-120. DOI: 10.14245/ns.1938454.227. Epub 2020 Mar 31

[24] Feizi N, Tavakoli M, Patel RV, Atashzar SF. Robotics and AI for teleoperation, tele-assessment, and tele-training for surgery in the era of COVID-19: Existing challenges, and future vision. Frontiers in Robotics and AI. 2021;**8**:610677. DOI: 10.3389/frobt.2021.610677

[25] Telesurgery Market – Top Key Players Competitive Scenario Study Report with Forecast by 2025 [Internet]. 2020. Available from: https://www.biospace.com/article/telesurgery-market-top-key-players-competitive-scenario-study-report-with-forecast-by-2025/ [Accessed: 2022-08-12]

[26] Haidegger T, Sándor J, Benyó Z. Surgery in space: The future of robotic telesurgery. Surgical Endoscopy. 2010;**25**(3):681-690

[27] Garcia P, Rosen J, Kapoor C, Noakes M, Elbert G, Treat M, et al. Trauma pod: A semi-automated Telerobotic surgical system. The International Journal of Medical Robotics and Computer Assisted Surgery. 2009;**5**(2):136-146

[28] Shin DH, Dalag L, Azhar RA, Santomauro M, Satkunasivam R, Metcalfe C, et al. A novel interface for the telementoring of robotic surgery. BJU International. 2015;**116**(2):302-308. DOI: 10.1111/bju.12985. Epub 2015 Mar 17

[29] Erridge S, Yeung DKT, Patel HRH, Purkayastha S. Telementoring of surgeons: A systematic review. Surgical Innovation. 2019;**26**(1):95-111. DOI: 10.1177/1553350618813250. Epub 2018 Nov 22

[30] Intuitive Announces First Quarter Earnings. Intuitive Surgical Available from: https://www.isrg.intuitive.com/news-releases/news-release-details/intuitive-announces-first-quarter-earnings-2. [Accessed: August 28, 2022]

[31] Patel S, Rovers MM, Sedelaar MJP, et al. How can robot-assisted surgery provide value for money? BMJ Surgery, Interventions, & Health Technologies. 2021;**3**:e000042. DOI: 10.1136/bmjsit-2020-000042

[32] Barbash GI, Glied SA. New technology and health care costs — The case of robot-assisted surgery. The New England Journal of Medicine Overseas Ed. 2010;**363**:701-704

[33] Marescaux J, Leroy J, Rubino F, Smith M, Vix M, Simone M, et al. Transcontinental robot-assisted remote telesurgery: Feasibility and potential applications. Annals of Surgery. 2002;**235**(4):487-492. DOI: 10.1097/00000658-200204000-00005

Section 3

The Far-Reaching Telehealth and Telemedicine on Services and Technologies

Chapter 7

Clinical Decision Support Systems for Diabetes Care: Evidence and Development between 2017 and Present

Xiaoni Zhang, Haoqiang Jiang and Gary Ozanich

Abstract

The clinical decision support systems (CDSs) for diabetes have improved significantly over the years. Multiple factors serve as driving forces for the uptake of CDSs. Newer technologies, initiatives, government mandates, and a competitive environment collectively facilitate advancement in diabetes care. This book chapter summarizes global CDSs development in recent years. Our review of the past few years' publications on CDSs for diabetes shows that the United States is leading the world in technology development and clinical evidence generation. Developing countries worldwide are catching up in CDSs development and standards of patient care. Though most CDSs and published studies are on diabetes diagnosis, treatment, and management, a small portion of the research is devoted to prediabetes and type I diabetes. Increased efforts worldwide have been devoted to artificial intelligence and machine learning in diabetes care.

Keywords: clinical decision support systems, diabetes care, machine learning, artificial intelligence, A1C, patient engagement, outcomes, clinical inertia

1. Introduction

Globally, chronic care conditions burden society with high costs and diminished quality of life for affected individuals. According to the Center for Disease Control and Prevention (CDC), more than one in 10 Americans ha diabetes mellitus, commonly referred to as type-2 diabetes (T2DM), and approximately one in three has prediabetes. Diabetes was the seventh leading cause of death in the United States in 2017. People with diagnosed diabetes, on average, have medical expenditures 2.3 times higher than those without diabetes [1], and 25% of all medical costs in the United States are spent on caring for people with diabetes. Diabetes can result in disabling complications, comorbidities, and reduced life expectancy. Effective management of diabetes is important to improve the quality of life for diabetics as well as improve population health and control medical costs. Attention and interventions are needed to address the issue of rising costs. Clinical decision support systems (CDSs) may offer the solution to rising costs, quality of care, patient engagement, patient-centered care, personalized medicine, clinical inertia, and clinical outcomes.

According to KBVResearch, the global CDSs market will grow from 2.9 billion in 2017 to 8.9 billion in 2027 [2]. The adoption of Electronic Health Record (EHR) and CDSs has been on the rise across the globe. Developed countries lead the development and implementation of CDSs. Several factors contribute to the increased acceptance and adoption of CDSs: general acceptance of using technologies across the entire healthcare spectrum, including adherence to clinical guidelines, evidence of improved clinic outcomes, government incentives, compliance/regulatory requirements, and operational efficiency. In this book chapter, we provide an overview of recent evidence on CDSs for diabetes care by searching relevant publications in CINAL, PsychInfo, Web of Science, Scopus, Medline, and PubMed from 2017 to the present.

2. Clinical decision support systems for diabetes care

2.1 Diabetes care

Diabetes is a chronic disease. Adequate diabetes care requires attention to biomarkers such as blood pressure, cholesterol, blood sugar level, and lifestyle changes. Care typically involves management of blood pressure, lipids, smoking, glucose, weight, screening for eye, foot, renal and vascular complications, and immunizations. It is common that patients with diabetes also have one or more other comorbid conditions. Thus, caring for diabetics is a team effort, and many providers may be involved, including various types of physicians or nurse practitioners, pharmacists, case managers, dieticians, and specialty doctors such as cardiologists, dentists, ophthalmologists, others. The literature has consistently reported a gap between current diabetes care practice and recommended diabetes care standards. This includes the concept of clinical inertia or the failure to start or accelerate a current or new therapy when appropriate. Clinical inertia may be due to the clinician's lack of knowledge or inexperience with new therapeutic interventions and drugs available to treat diabetes [3].

Many IT-based interventions have been developed to improve adherence to the quality of care standards for chronic illnesses such as diabetes. CDSs for diabetes have been developed to address prediabetes screening, type I, type II, and gestational diabetes diagnosis, treatment, and care. **Figure 1** shows the publications related to CDSs in diabetes. Though CDSs predated EHR, it is well documented in the literature that the adoption of CDSs is low [4].

2.2 Clinical decision support (CDS)

A clinical decision support (CDS) is a computerized system that uses case-based reasoning to assist clinicians in various decision-making such as assessing disease status, diagnosis, selecting appropriate therapy, or making other clinical decisions [5]. CDSs are typically used at the point of care where clinicians can make treatment decisions either based on their own knowledge or by combining their knowledge with patient characteristics or recommendations provided by the CDS through a clinical disease-specific knowledge base. CDSs provide alerts, reminders, or feedback to a care team [6]. A CDS can improve healthcare delivery by improving medical decisions with targeted clinical knowledge, patient information, and other health information [7].

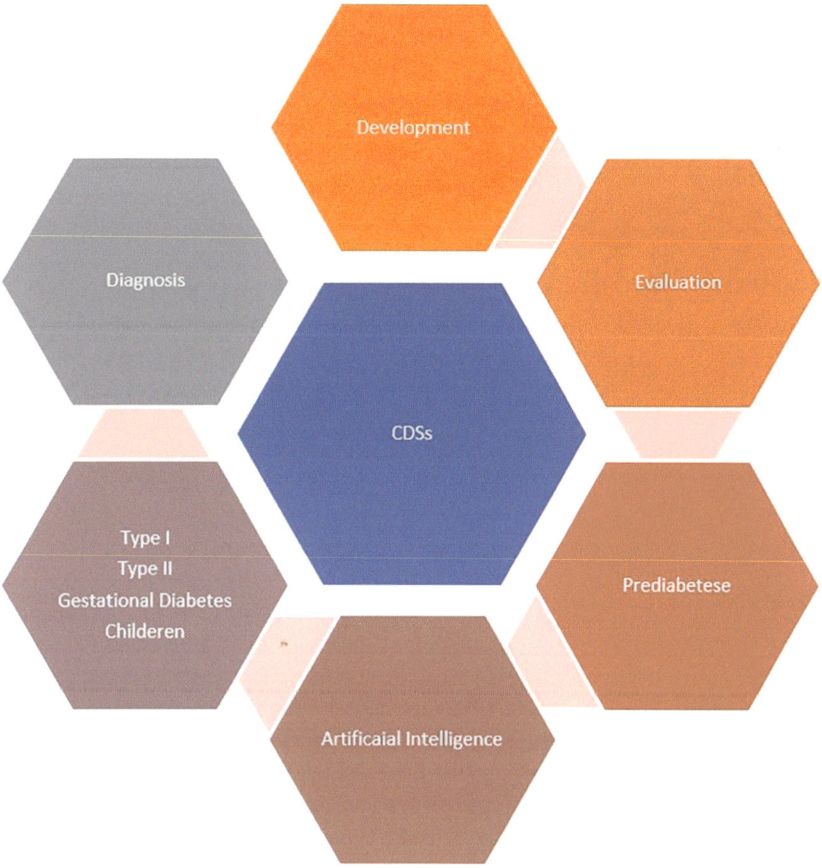

Figure 1.
CDSs research areas.

2.2.1 History of clinical decision support

The idea was generated in the 1950s. In the late 1960s, F. T. deDombal and his associates at the University of Leeds studied the diagnostic process. They developed the Leeds abdominal pain system, a computer-based decision aid using Bayesian probability theory to explain seven possible causes of acute abdominal pain. In the 1970s, Stanford University developed MYCIN, rule-based decision support using a reasonably simple inference engine and a knowledge base of 600 rules. Later, Help was developed, and both MYCIN and HELP could generate alerts when abnormal factors were observed. Earlier studies on CDSs report that the use of automated clinical guidelines for diabetes in general practice did not result in a clinically significant change in doctors' behavior or in patient outcomes [8].

2.2.2 Components of CDSs

Figure 2 depicts the components of a CDS. Typically, a CDS consists of a knowledge base, inference engine, and communication mechanism. The knowledge base contains facts, best practices, clinical guidelines or protocols, drug interactions, drug allergies, and logical rules. The inference engine combines patient-specific data

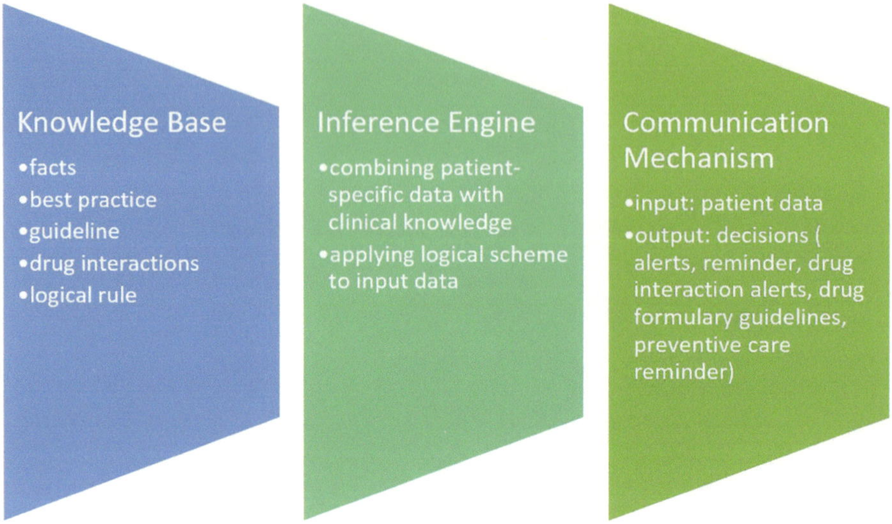

Figure 2.
Components of CDSs.

(demographic data, medical history, family history) with clinical knowledge and performs reasoning. The communication mechanism takes patient data as input and produces output including alerts, reminders, summaries, etc.

Different technologies are used to build CDSs. Some use open-source software. For example, Protégé and WebProtégé are free software programs for building ontology knowledge solutions, and Jena is the Java rule-based inference engine. WebProtégé builds drug knowledge, and Jena evaluates the antidiabetic medications reasoning module [9].

2.3 Benefits of clinical decision support systems in diabetes

Digital transformation involves fundamentally rethinking healthcare delivery processes, treatments, and services from a technology-enabled perspective. CDSs promote diabetes care by facilitating evidence-informed insulin use, improving blood glucose control, and quality indicators in caring for patients with diabetes. Given the complex undertaking for clinicians, CDSs may simplify and improve the care process and patient outcomes. CDSs could be valuable when delivering medical care to better match patients' preferences and biological characteristics. Normally, CDSs automatically provide specific treatment recommendations.

Commercial developers typically promote CDSs to improve clinical decision-making, reduce medication errors and misdiagnoses, provide consistent and reliable information, enhance operational efficiency, increase patient satisfaction, improve quality of care, and lower costs. The literature echoes some of the claims made by these vendors. For example, a systematic review suggests that CDSs reduce unwarranted practice variation, improve healthcare quality, reduce waste in the healthcare system, and decrease the risk of overload and burnout among clinicians [10]. Some devoted efforts to developing a user-friendly, comprehensive, fully integrated web and mobile-based clinical decision support and monitoring system for the screening, diagnosis, treatment, and monitoring of diabetes [11].

2.3.1 Outcomes

Recent studies show positive outcomes in controlling glucose levels for patients with diabetes. A CDS was associated with improving the comprehensive control of blood pressure, LDLc, and HbA1c for diabetics in primary care [12]. Glucose Path, an AI-enabled CDSs for diabetes, effectively reduces the glucose level of patients with poorly controlled diabetes in the Medicaid population. These CDSs facilitate team-based care allowing a cost-effective solution to be produced for patients [13]. GlycASSIST, another diabetes CDS, facilitated treatment intensification and was acceptable to patients with diabetes and general practitioners [14]. A CDS tool on the management of diabetes in small- to medium-sized primary care practices participating in Delaware's patient-centered medical home project finds the use of CDS is correlated with greater reductions from baseline in hemoglobin A1c and low-density lipoprotein cholesterol, and more patients achieving treatment goals, aiding physicians and staff in better clinical decision-making [15]. EHR CDS was successful in reducing hyperglycemic events among hospitalized patients with dysglycemia and diabetes and inappropriate insulin use in patients with type 1 diabetes [16].

2.3.2 Clinician satisfaction

Additional studies have found clinician satisfaction with CDSs use in treating diabetes and facilitating treatment intensification by the general practitioners [14]. In a cluster-randomized trial, an EHR-linked, web-based CDSs significantly improved glucose and blood pressure control in diabetes patients. The CDS has high use rate and clinician satisfaction. As a result, users are willing to recommend the CDS to others [17]. Furthermore, recent evidence shows that the majority of physicians are satisfied with CDSs [18]. The CDS was feasible and acceptable to GPs [19].

2.3.3 Operational efficiency

CDS for diabetes can help with disease management, and its web-based system CDS provides on-time registration, reports of diabetic prevalence, uncontrolled diabetes, and diabetic complications and reduces the rate of mismanagement of diabetes [20]. In a qualitative evaluation of a standalone CDSs for medication reminders, CDSs were found to improve adherence to evidence-based guidelines and support a more efficient ordering process for providers; providers are satisfied with the CDS for diabetes [21]. CDSs improve healthcare professionals' adherence to suggested insulin doses and workflow tasks. The decision support system facilitates safe and efficacious inpatient diabetes care by standardizing treatment workflow and providing decision support for basal-bolus insulin dosing [22]. The CDSs integrated with the Epic EHR at the University of Utah enable clinicians and patients to review relevant patient parameters, select treatment goals, and review alternate treatment strategies based on prediction results. The proposed analytical method outperformed previous machine-learning algorithms on prediction accuracy [23].

2.4 Barriers

Despite the benefits documented in the literature, there are barriers to using CDSs. Prior studies suggest time and reimbursement [15], interference with established workflow, unhelpful or irrelevant recommendations, and time pressures [24]. In practice, time constraints, patient overpopulation, and complex guidelines require alternative solutions for real-time patient monitoring. Physician guidelines use rates for diagnosis, treatment, and monitoring of diabetes are very low. To successfully implement a CDS, organizations must conduct adequate validation of programs, evidence and knowledge-based assimilation, users' feedback, widespread implementation in collaboration with stakeholders, and consistent evaluation of programs' impact [16]. In order for the CDSs to be effective, the CDS should be conceived as part of a broader, coherent, and department-wide quality improvement strategy, where a clinical quality gap between current patient outcomes or processes and the desired end state has been clearly identified and carefully measured.

3. Global overview of CDSs

This section covers the global development of CDSs; two subsections are created to highlight leading CDSs in industrialized countries and developing countries on technological infrastructure, practice habits, and patient expectations.

3.1 Industrialized countries

In Europe, C3-Cloud is a European Union's initiative to implement digital health Europe; it is a multinational effort for integrated patient-centered care in the co-occurrence of chronic diseases. C3-Cloud has a group of 12 partners across seven countries in Europe. The care for patients with multiple chronic conditions is complex; it is common that patient data are located across multiple systems and in silos; it is difficult to get a complete, accurate, and reliable view of patients' medical history. C3-Cloud project aims to build an integrated care platform, so clinicians have better and complete patient information to make clinical decisions; such systems address the increasing demand for improved health outcomes of patients with multiple chronic conditions.

In addition to C3-Cloud addressing multiple chronic conditions, the MOSAIC project in European Union particularly focuses on decision support for diabetes; this project takes a participatory development approach; it applies persuasive design techniques and business modeling to define three phases: (1) user needs, (2) system implementation, and (3) evaluation of the use of CDSs in diabetes management. Qualitative studies using focus groups were used to compile system requirements to gain new insights in the definition of effective Decision Support Systems to deal with the complexity of diabetes care [25].

Several countries (Turkey, Spain, the United Kingdom, Sweden, Finland, and France) collaborated and developed an ICT infrastructure with guidelines to enable personalized care plan management for addressing the needs of patients with multi-morbidity. The team designed 43 logical flowcharts of four disease guidelines (Type 2 Diabetes, Heart Failure, Renal Failure, and Depression) and implemented 181 CDS rules [26].

In Italy, a multidisciplinary research team consisting of doctors, clinicians, and IT engineers develop a fuzzy inference machine to improve the quality of the day-to-day clinical care of type-2 diabetic patients at the Anti-Diabetes Center. This CDS has the function of remote patient monitoring, which includes the ability to monitor a patient regularly from home. This may help to reduce hospitalizations or other acute events [27].

In Belgium, a cluster-randomized trial with before-and-after measurements of a CDS was conducted in Belgian Primary Care Practices over 1 year between May 2017 and May 2018. The majority of physicians were satisfied with the EBMeDS system. Clinicians report many benefits of using CDS, including rapid access to (patient-specific) drug interactions, problems, evidence-based links, etc. Clinicians do not need to perform extensive searching for guidelines. On the disadvantage side, clinicians mention the time required to use the system, the increased alertness by the system, and incorrect reminders. The clinical trial concluded that EBMeDS did not improve diabetes care in Belgian primary care despite the benefits. However, this trial has a significant drop-out rate of 43%. This high drop rate may weaken the conclusion drawn from this study. Further analysis shows the lack of improvement was mainly caused by inadequate software training, EHR data transfer issues, auto coding of lab results, and technical and reporting issues [18].

Another study on CDS for diabetes in Belgium tackles the inappropriate tests as they are a waste of healthcare resources with a pragmatic, cluster-randomized, open-label, controlled clinical trial. This CDS is integrated into a computerized physician order entry (CPOE) to examine the appropriateness and volume of laboratory test ordering and diagnostic errors in primary care. The results show that a CDS within the CPOE improves the appropriateness of lab tests and decreases the volume of laboratory test ordering without increasing diagnostic error [28].

In Saudi Arabia, an evaluation study of EHR integrated CDS reports no significant improvement in chronic disease outcomes [29]. In South Korea, a CDS for Diabetes was developed based on the innovative integration of ontology and fuzzy-ruled reasoning with real data sets. This CDS has an open architecture that is scalable, extensible and increases accuracy in diagnosing diabetes [30].

In Taiwan, a CDS with a focus on antidiabetic medication recommendations was developed based on the guidelines of the American Diabetes Association and the European Association for the study of diabetes. The CDS enables doctors' clinical diagnosis and decision-making for specialty physicians, nonspecialty doctors, and young doctors with their drug prescriptions. The physician evaluation of the system shows that 87% think the system is useful, and 85% are satisfied with the CDS in their care of diabetes patient [9].

In Australia, a prototype (GlycASSIST) is integrated into an electronic medical record containing evidence-based guidelines. GlycASSIST helps general practice and patients during encounters for setting glycated hemoglobin (HbA1c) targets and intensifying treatment. Interviews and focus groups are conducted with clinicians, including four General Practices, five endocrinologists, three diabetes educators, and six patients with type 2 diabetes. Clinicians and people with diabetes believe that GlycASSIST is useful in individualized treatment intensification. They recommended that GlycASSIST enhances the visual appeal and allows clinicians to overwrite recommendations. In addition, clinicians requested CDS be easily navigated and have greater prescribing guidance [14].

In Turkey, a web and mobile-based application will be developed, which allows the physician to remotely monitor patient data through mobile applications in real time. This system will perform the function of screening, diagnosis, treatment, and monitoring of diabetes diseases. The developed CDS will be tested in two stages: first, the usability, understandability, and adequacy of the application will be determined. Second, a parallel, single-blind, randomized controlled trial will be implemented. Diabetes-diagnosed patients will be recruited for the CDS trial by their primary care physicians [11]. GlycASSIST was able to achieve its purpose of facilitating treatment intensification and was acceptable to people with T2D and GPs. The GlycASSIST prototype is being refined based on these findings to prepare for quantitative evaluation [14].

In Canada, a CDS assists primary care practitioners in applying standardized behavior change strategies and clinical practice guidelines-based recommendations to an individual patient and empowers the patient with the skills and knowledge required to self-manage their diabetes through planned, personalized, and pervasive behavior change strategies. A qualitative study was then conducted to evaluate usability, functionality, usefulness, and acceptance [31].

In summary, CDSs developed in industrialized countries typically incorporate evidence-based practice into the design and development. The commonly followed guidelines are either published by American Diabetes Association or the European Association. Recent findings report a more positive user experience with CDSs, user acceptance, operational efficiency, and clinical outcomes.

3.2 CDSs in developing countries

Developing countries face far greater challenges and barriers than industrialized countries managing chronic diseases. Economic backgrounds, lack of resources, and the absence of some laboratory tests may make clinical guidelines published by international associations not applicable to developing countries. In Sri Lanka, about 11% of its total population has diabetes [32]. A CDS for diabetes was developed through two stages: first, mapping the diabetes-related clinical guidelines using the business process model and notation 2.0 for type 1 and type 2 diabetes and gestational diabetes; second, treatment plans were developed with guidelines using flowcharting. Domain experts were consulted to design and evaluate the ontology. Several real-life diabetic scenarios are used to validate and evaluate the ontology [33].

In Egypt, data mining techniques were used to develop classifiers for the early diagnosis of diabetes. An ensemble algorithm significantly outperforms all other classifiers. Such an effort is essential in building a personalized decision support system, aiding physicians in their daily clinical practice [34].

In Iran, a web-based CDS for diabetes diagnosis and management was developed using ASP.Net MVC server technology, Razor engine, SQL Server database, HTML 5, CSS 3 world standard, and Ajax technology. The diabetes CDS is built following the American Diabetes Association and American Association of Clinical Endocrinologists (AACE) guidelines and physical activity 2017 guidelines recommended by the Netherland. Its interface is user-friendliness and easy to use. The interface displays demographic data, past medical history, laboratory tests, lifestyle, and family history. The web-based system allows for on-time registration, better reporting on diabetic status (uncontrolled diabetes, diabetic complications), and reducing the rate of mismanagement of diabetes. It helps the physicians in managing the patients more effectively [20].

In India, the cost of early diagnosis of diabetes is a barrier for many people to get the laboratory testing done. Various machine learning algorithms are integrated with a CDS to assess diabetes [35].

In summary, developing countries have improved their technological development in patient care. However, evidence-based guidelines are not consistently incorporated into the design of CDSs. Interestingly, developing countries explore data mining and machine learning in an innovative way. Algorithms and predictive models are developed to predict prediabetes and diabetes without any lab tests.

Predictive models could not be 100% accurate. Clinicians and data scientists need to work together to determine the acceptable level for model performance. There will be some false positive or false negative. Data scientists need to work with clinicians to determine the pros and cons of false positive and false negative. In the area of prediabetes, false positive may not produce detrimental effect than false positive. Then the models that produce false positive may be more acceptable than false.

4. Machine learning and artificial intelligence negative

Artificial intelligence (AI) allows computers to describe, understand, learn, reason, and integrate information to solve problems. AI simulates human intelligence so that better, quicker decisions can be made. AI is a fast-growing field utilized by many medical areas, enabling computers to gain human-like intelligence. For example, its applications to diabetes, a global pandemic, can change and improve the approach to diagnosis and management of diabetes. AI is useful in specialized CDSs for detecting diabetic retinopathy [36]. AI revolutionizes remote patient monitoring, continuously monitors the patient's symptoms and biomarkers, and adjusts to medicine and treatment in real-time, resulting in better clinical outcomes, including glycemic control with reductions in fasting and postprandial glucose levels, glucose excursions, and glycosylated hemoglobin. AI will reform conventional diabetes care by using a targeted data-driven approach and personalized care [37]. However, in regard to user attitudes, a survey study finds that negative perceptions of AI-based CDS tools may reduce staff excitement about AI technology [36]. Thus, it is important to have hands-on experience with AI so that users can gain more realistic expectations about the technology's capabilities.

Machine learning (ML) is a subset of AI. Machine learning features that machines can learn over time without being explicitly programmed. The ML algorithms include decision trees, random forests, artificial neural networks, genetic algorithms, and support vector machines. The ML algorithms have been used in building predictive risk models for diabetes or its consequent complications. For example, a web-based CDS can predict the early-stage risk of diabetes by classifying results using the patient's questionnaire without a testing kit. This CDS applies a deep learning approach resulting in better prediction accuracy than supervised machine learning [38]. Another study finds that fuzzy inference machines improve the quality of the day-by-day clinical care of diabetic patients and allow the remote monitoring of patients' clinical conditions, which helps to reduce hospitalizations [27].

Though AI seems to have unlimited possibilities, there are challenges to the adoption of diabetes AI devices, apps, and systems. Factors such as costs, user acceptance, physician cooperation, and interoperability between systems may affect how an innovation is adopted [39].

5. Future care for diabetes

Medical futurists predict there will be a cure for diabetes. A recent study on stem cells also concludes that beta cell replacement holds a promising cure for diabetes [36]. Biological and medical breakthroughs like the artificial pancreas, and glucose-responsive insulin, provide the correct insulin and the right time to patients. Regarding patient care in diabetes, virtual doctors, big data, data analytics, and social media, all these will become intertwined in the entire patient care ecosystem. Virtual doctors, a proof-of-concept CDS powered by an AI speech recognition system, are able to interact with patients and predict diabetes based on noninvasive sensors and deep neural networks [40]. Wearable technologies enable individualized monitoring of physiological variables in real time. The real-time data collected from multiple devices combined are fed into an artificial intelligence model using adaptive-neuro fuzzy interference to detect prediabetes and diabetes [41].

There is no doubt that digital transformation in healthcare will continue. Big data, machine learning, artificial intelligence, EHR-integrated, web-based, and mobile apps will improve, enhance, and adopt diabetes care. Medical and consumer devices collect a vast amount and variety of data, including continuous glucose monitoring data, insulin pump data, heart rate, hours of sleep, the number of steps walked, movement captured by wristbands or watches, hydration, geolocation, and barometric pressure. Next-generation developments of CDS will leverage big data and prioritize clinical actions based on data analysis, delivering maximum benefits to a given patient at the point of care. In the meantime, innovative care models and delivery methods will emerge. Personalized medication recommendations offered by CDSs fit each patient's insurance coverage, budget, lifestyle, and medicines. Outcomes can be analyzed constantly and regularly so that adjustments to medicines can be targeted based on the most recent patients' biological data.

Early diagnosis of diabetes and treatment will reduce the risk of developing comorbidity, delay the development of comorbidity, and improve quality of life for patients. CDSs facilitate doctors in clinical diagnosis and overcome clinical inertia in terms of prescribing habits. In addition, patient-centered care should consider patients' preferences in care decisions and identify effective methods to communicate CDS information to patients. Doctors need to be more tech-savvy in learning the latest technologies on patient care; patients want more empowerment by participating in self-care and care decision-making. Furthermore, increased number of diabetes journals publish AI-related technologies in diabetes care. Now, doctors must learn new skills and knowledge on AI tools, which have become part of diabetes health care [42].

A path forward may be computerized virtual coaches replacing human counseling; virtual doctors will be able to fully engage in the diagnosis, treatment, and continuous monitoring of chronic diseases. CDSs can be as good or superior to human doctors when prescribing diabetes medicines and may be more effective in overcoming clinical inertia as CDSs can remove human biases and habits. Considering the fact that the physician shortage is growing and 10.5% of the population has diabetes, CDSs play an important role in treating diabetes and more efficiently using clinical resources [43].

6. Conclusion

The CDSs for diabetes have improved significantly over the years. Multiple factors serve as driving forces for the uptake of CDSs. Newer technologies, initiatives, government mandates, and a competitive environment collectively facilitate advancement in diabetes care. This book chapter summarizes global CDSs development in recent years. Our review of the past few years' publications on CDSs for diabetes shows that the United States is leading the world in technology development and clinical evidence generation. Developing countries around the world are catching up in CDSs development and standards of patient care. The literature has consistently documented evidence of operational efficiency delivered by CDSs (e.g., reduced medical errors and reduced duplicate tests). The current evidence shows that both developing and industrialized countries have put more effort into AI and ML and will use artificial intelligence to their own advantage and innovative ways to develop more sophisticated diabetes CDS tools.

Though studies conducted 5 years prior commonly reported a low adoption rate of CDSs [4], recent publications show an increase in the adoption of CDSs, especially if CDSs are integrated into workflow and EHR. Our recent study of a quality improvement project using Glucose Pathway confirms this trend. In our project, the vendor has been working on integration with EHR. With the increased integration of CDSs with EHR, CDS adoption and utilization will significantly increase. CDS' true and long-term impact on outcomes, safety, and cost savings can be better measured and validated.

Advancements in technologies will continue to transform patient care, including doctors, processes, and patients. All entities in the patient engagement systems must learn, adapt, and adopt new developments to achieve better self-care, patient care, and clinical decisions. The future is bright but demands more learning on technologies.

Conflict of interest

The authors declare no conflict of interest.

Author details

Xiaoni Zhang[1,2*], Haoqiang Jiang[1] and Gary Ozanich[1]

1 Northern Kentucky University, Highland Heights, KY, USA

2 The University of Alabama at Birmingham, Birmingham, AL, USA

*Address all correspondence to: xzhang2@uab.edu

References

[1] Association AD. Economic costs of diabetes in the US in 2017. Diabetes Care. 2018;**41**(5):917-928

[2] Global Clinical Decision Support Systems Market Size, Share & Industry Trends Analysis Report By Component, By Product, By Delivery Mode, By Application, By Regional Outlook, Strategy, Challenges and Forecast, 2021-2027, 2022. Available from: https://www.kbvresearch.com/clinical-decision-support-systems-market/. [Accessed: May 13, 2022]

[3] Khunti K, Gomes MB, Pocock S, Shestakova MV, Pintat S, Fenici P, et al. Therapeutic inertia in the treatment of hyperglycaemia in patients with type 2 diabetes: A systematic review. Diabetes, Obesity and Metabolism. 2018;**20**(2):427-437. DOI: 10.1111/dom.13088

[4] Ali SM, Giordano R, Lakhani S, Walker DM. A review of randomized controlled trials of medical record powered clinical decision support system to improve quality of diabetes care. International Journal of Medical Informatics. 2016;**87**:91-100. DOI: 10.1016/j.ijmedinf.2015.12.017

[5] Osheroff JA, Teich JM, Middleton B, Steen EB, Wright A, Detmer DE. A roadmap for national action on clinical decision support. Journal of the American Medical Informatics Association. 2007;**14**(2):141-145. DOI: 10.1197/jamia.m2334

[6] Jia W, Zhang P, Duolikun N, Zhu D, Li H, Bao Y. Study protocol for the road to hierarchical diabetes management at primary care (ROADMAP) study in China: A cluster randomised controlled trial. BMJ Open. 2020;**10**(1):e032734. DOI: 10.1136/bmjopen-2019-032734

[7] Osheroff JA, Teich JM, Levick D, Saldana L, Velasco FT, Sittig DF. Improving Outcomes with Clinical Decision Support: An Implementer's Guide. Chicago, IL: Himss Publishing; 2012

[8] Hetlevik I, Holmen J, Krüger Ø, Kristensen P, Iversen H, Furuseth K. Implementing clinical guidelines in the treatment of diabetes mellitus in general practice: Evaluation of effort, process, and patient outcome related to implementation of a computer-based decision support system. International Journal of Technology Assessment in Health Care. 2000;**16**(1):210-227. DOI: 10.1080/028134399750002872

[9] Chen R-C, Jiang HQ, Huang C-Y, Bau C-T. Clinical decision support system for diabetes based on ontology reasoning and TOPSIS analysis. Journal of Healthcare Engineering. 2017:2017. DOI: 10.1155/2017/4307508

[10] Hunt DL, Haynes RB, Hanna SE, Smith K. Effects of computer-based clinical decision support systems on physician performance and patient outcomes: A systematic review. Journal of the American Medical Association. 1998;**280**(15):1339-1346. DOI: 10.1001/jama.280.15.1339

[11] Kart Ö, Mevsim V, Kut A, Yürek İ, Altın AÖ, Yılmaz O. A mobile and web-based clinical decision support and monitoring system for diabetes mellitus patients in primary care: A study protocol for a randomized controlled trial. BMC Medical Informatics and Decision Making. 2017;**17**(1):1-10. DOI: 10.1186/s12911-017-0558-6

[12] Beltrán LM, Olmo-Fernández A, Banegas JR, García-Puig J. Electronic clinical decision support system and

multifactorial risk factor control in patients with type 2 diabetes in primary health care. European Journal of Internal Medicine. 2017;**44**:e35-ee7. DOI: 10.1016/j.ejim.2017.07.024

[13] Zhang X, Svec M, Tracy R, Ozanich G. Clinical decision support systems with team-based care on type 2 diabetes improvement for Medicaid patients: A quality improvement project. International Journal of Medical Informatics. 2022;**158**:104626. DOI: 10.1016/j.ijmedinf.2021.104626

[14] Kunstler BE, Furler J, Holmes-Truscott E, McLachlan H, Boyle D, Lo S, et al. Guiding glucose management discussions among adults with type 2 diabetes in general practice: Development and pretesting of a clinical decision support tool prototype embedded in an electronic medical record. JMIR Formative Research. 2020;**4**(9):e17785. DOI: 10.2196/17785

[15] Gill J, Kucharski K, Turk B, Pan C, Wei W. Using electronic clinical decision support in patient-centered medical homes to improve management of diabetes in primary care: The DECIDE study. The Journal of Ambulatory Care Management. 2019;**42**(2):105. DOI: 10.1097/jac.0000000000000267

[16] Pichardo-Lowden A, Umpierrez G, Lehman EB, Bolton MD, DeFlitch CJ, Chinchilli VM, et al. Clinical decision support to improve management of diabetes and dysglycemia in the hospital: A path to optimizing practice and outcomes. BMJ Open Diabetes Research and Care. 2021;**9**(1):e001557. DOI: 10.1136/bmjdrc-2020-001557

[17] Sperl-Hillen JM, Rossom RC, Kharbanda EO, Gold R, Geissal ED, Elliott TE, et al. Priorities wizard: Multisite web-based primary care clinical decision support improved chronic care outcomes with high use rates and high clinician satisfaction rates. eGEMs. 2019;**7**(1). DOI: 10.5334/egems.284

[18] Heselmans A, Delvaux N, Laenen A, Van de Velde S, Ramaekers D, Kunnamo I, et al. Computerized clinical decision support system for diabetes in primary care does not improve quality of care: A cluster-randomized controlled trial. Implementation Science. 2020;**15**(1):1-14. DOI: 10.1186/s13012-019-0955-6

[19] Murphy ME, McSharry J, Byrne M, Boland F, Corrigan D, Gillespie P, et al. Supporting care for suboptimally controlled type 2 diabetes mellitus in general practice with a clinical decision support system: A mixed methods pilot cluster randomised trial. BMJ Open. 2020;**10**(2):e032594. DOI: 10.1136/bmjopen-2019-032594

[20] Johari MG, Dabaghmanesh M, Zare H, Safaeian A, Abdollahifard G. Smart diabetic screening and managing software, a novel decision support system. Journal of Biomedical Physics & Engineering. 2018;**8**(3):289. DOI: 10.31661/jbpe.v8i3sep.870

[21] Larsen K, Akindele B, Head H, Evans R, Mehta P, Hlatky Q, et al. Developing a user-centered digital clinical decision support app for evidence-based medication recommendations for Type 2 diabetes mellitus: Prototype user testing and validation study. JMIR Human Factors. 2022;**9**(1):e33470. DOI: 10.2196/33470

[22] Lichtenegger KM, Aberer F, Tuca AC, Donsa K, Höll B, Schaupp L, et al. Safe and sufficient glycemic control by using a digital clinical decision support system for patients with type 2 diabetes in a routine setting on general hospital wards. Journal of Diabetes Science and

Technology. 2021;**15**(2):231-235. DOI: 10.1177/1932296820955243

[23] Tarumi S, Takeuchi W, Chalkidis G, Rodriguez-Loya S, Kuwata J, Flynn M, et al. Leveraging artificial intelligence to improve chronic disease care: Methods and application to pharmacotherapy decision support for type-2 diabetes mellitus. Methods of Information in Medicine. 2021;**60**(S 01):e32-e43. DOI: 10.1055/s-0041-1728757

[24] Khairat S, Marc D, Crosby W, Al SA. Reasons for physicians not adopting clinical decision support systems: Critical analysis. JMIR Medical Informatics. 2018;**6**(2):e8912. DOI: 10.2196/medinform.8912

[25] Fico G, Hernanzez L, Cancela J, Dagliati A, Sacchi L, Martinez-Millana A, et al. What do healthcare professionals need to turn risk models for type 2 diabetes into usable computerized clinical decision support systems? Lessons learned from the MOSAIC project. BMC Medical Informatics and Decision Making. 2019;**19**(1):1-16. DOI: 10.1186/s12911-019-0887-8

[26] Laleci Erturkmen GB, Yuksel M, Sarigul B, Lindman P, Chen R, Zhao L, et al. Management of personalised guideline-driven care plans addressing the needs of multi-morbidity via clinical decision support services. International Journal of Integrated Care. 2018: University of Utrecht. DOI: 10.5334/ijic.s2132

[27] Ylenia C, Giovanni I, Lucia R, Donatella V, Tiziana S, Vincenzo G, et al. A clinical decision support system based on fuzzy rules and classification algorithms for monitoring the physiological parameters of type-2 diabetic patients. Mathematical Biosciences and Engineering. 2021;**18**(3):2654-2674. DOI: 10.3934/mbe.2021135

[28] Delvaux N, Piessens V, Burghgraeve TD, Mamouris P, Vaes B, Stichele RV, et al. Clinical decision support improves the appropriateness of laboratory test ordering in primary care without increasing diagnostic error: The ELMO cluster randomized trial. Implementation Science. 2020;**15**(1):1-10. DOI: 10.1186/s13012-020-01059-y

[29] Mahmoud AS, Alkhenizan A, Shafiq M, Alsoghayer S. The impact of the implementation of a clinical decision support system on the quality of healthcare services in a primary care setting. Journal of Family Medicine and Primary Care. 2020;**9**(12):6078. DOI: 10.4103/jfmpc.jfmpc_1728_20

[30] El-Sappagh S, Alonso JM, Ali F, Ali A, Jang J-H, Kwak K-S. An ontology-based interpretable fuzzy decision support system for diabetes diagnosis. IEEE Access. 2018;**6**:37371-37394. DOI: 10.1109/ACCESS.2018.2852004

[31] Abidi S, Vallis M, Piccinini-Vallis H, Imran SA, Abidi SSR. Diabetes-related behavior change knowledge transfer to primary care practitioners and patients: Implementation and evaluation of a digital health platform. JMIR Medical Informatics. 2018;**6**(2):e9629. DOI: 10.2196/medinform.9629

[32] Diabetes prevalence in Sri Lanka. 2021. Available from: https://data.worldbank.org/indicator/SH.STA.DIAB.ZS?end=2021&locations=LK&start=2021. [Accessed: May 25, 2022]

[33] Madhusanka S, Walisadeera A, Dantanarayana G, Goonetillake J, Ginige A, editors. An ontological clinical decision support system based on clinical guidelines for diabetes patients in Sri Lanka. Healthcare. Multidisciplinary Digital Publishing Institute. 2020;**8**(4):573. DOI: 10.3390/healthcare8040573

[34] El-Sappagh S, Elmogy M, Ali F, Abuhmed T, Islam S, Kwak K-S. A comprehensive medical decision–support framework based on a heterogeneous ensemble classifier for diabetes prediction. Electronics. 2019;**8**(6):635. DOI: 10.3390/electronics8060635

[35] Ramanujam E, Chandrakumar T, Thivyadharsine K, Varsha D, editors. A multilingual decision support system for early detection of diabetes using machine learning approach: Case study for Rural Indian people. In: 2020 Fifth International Conference on Research in Computational Intelligence and Communication Networks (ICRCICN). Bangalore, India: IEEE; 2020. DOI: 10.1109/icrcicn50933.2020.9296187

[36] Bourgeois S, Sawatani T, Van Mulders A, De Leu N, Heremans Y, Heimberg H, et al. Towards a functional cure for diabetes using stem cell-derived beta cells: Are we there yet? Cell. 2021;**10**(1):191. DOI: 10.3390/cells10010191

[37] Ellahham S. Artificial intelligence: The future for diabetes care. The American Journal of Medicine. 2020;**133**(8):895-900. DOI: 10.1016/j.amjmed.2020.03.033

[38] Pankaj C, Singh KV, Singh KR, editors. Artificial intelligence enabled web-based prediction of diabetes using machine learning approach. In: 2021 International Conference on Disruptive Technologies for Multi-Disciplinary Research and Applications (CENTCON). IEEE; 2021. DOI: 10.1109/CENTCON52345.2021.9688236

[39] Dankwa-Mullan I, Rivo M, Sepulveda M, Park Y, Snowdon J, Rhee K. Transforming diabetes care through artificial intelligence: The future is here. Population Health Management. 2019;**22**(3):229-242. DOI: 10.1089/pop.2018.0129

[40] Spänig S, Emberger-Klein A, Sowa J-P, Canbay A, Menrad K, Heider D. The virtual doctor: An interactive clinical-decision-support system based on deep learning for non-invasive prediction of diabetes. Artificial Intelligence in Medicine. 2019;**100**:101706. DOI: 10.1016/j.artmed.2019.101706

[41] Baig MM, GholamHosseini H, Moqeem AA, Mirza F, Lindén M. Clinical decision support systems in hospital care using ubiquitous devices: Current issues and challenges. Health Informatics Journal. 2019;**25**(3):1091-1104. DOI: 10.1177/1460458217740722

[42] Rigla M, García-Sáez G, Pons B, Hernando ME. Artificial intelligence methodologies and their application to diabetes. Journal of Diabetes Science and Technology. 2018;**12**(2):303-310. DOI: 10.1177/1932296817710475

[43] National Diabetes Statistics Report 2020. Available from: https://www.cdc.gov/diabetes/library/features/diabetes-stat-report.html. [Accessed: May 29, 2021]

Chapter 8

Application of Systemic Accident Analysis (SAA) Approaches in Telemedicine/Telehealth

Oseghale Igene and Aimee Ferguson

Abstract

This chapter discusses the importance of applying methods based on the systems thinking paradigm in analysing accidents that may occur in a complex healthcare system involving telemedicine/telehealth. Different accident analysis approaches (models and methods) have been utilised to analyse incidents/accidents in different safety-critical domains, including healthcare, to identify weaknesses and to be able to propose safety recommendations. With the advent of systemic accident analysis (SAA) approaches based on the systems thinking paradigm, can they be feasibly and practically applied to incidents resulting from unintended issues relating to telemedicine/telehealth? This chapter discusses three popular SAA approaches, benefits and limitations, including their necessity for improving safety and even security relating to telemedicine processes.

Keywords: AcciMap, STAMP, safety, security, healthcare

1. Introduction

Telemedicine/telehealth are terms often used interchangeably to describe the use of digital technologies to provide healthcare services remotely [1]. It comprises a diverse collection of technologies (e.g., telephone, video, software, apps, instant messaging, email, online forms) and clinical applications (e.g., providing routine consultations remotely; monitoring patients at home; remote consultations, remote monitoring of symptoms, robotic surgery with a surgeon in another location). Most operational telemedicine processes/services that focus on diagnosis and clinical management remotely are carried out in industrialised countries (e.g., USA, Canada, United Kingdom, and Australia). Telemedicine has provided benefits for both patients and healthcare professionals. For patients, this includes better access to healthcare, including primary care (communication with GP and home monitoring) and secondary care (emergency specialist support, intra & inter-hospital access, shared case for diagnosis and treatment) [2], especially if they live rurally, and may be unable to attend to ill health or other commitments (e.g., work, caring). For healthcare professionals, telemedicine allows them to connect with other clinical specialists/ colleagues to assist with consultations regarding a patient. Telemedicine is also expected and helps to improve the quality of care, equity of healthcare access and delivery efficiency in this regard [3]. The two main reasons telemedicine is utilised is because there is no alternative to this process, and it is considered better than conventional healthcare services [3].

Heinzeleman, Lugan and Kvedar noted in their paper that the future of telemedicine depended on three major aspects, including human factors, economic factors and technology [4]. Human factors comprise behaviours relating to how technology influences existing policies, culture, knowledge, and attitudes which can fundamentally affect changes at different levels in a complex socio-technical system like healthcare [4]. These levels consist of individual, organisational and societal levels. Individuals include patients who appreciate and expect high-quality, technology-enabled healthcare and healthcare providers (where their perceptions and behaviours are considered very important). At the organisational level, there is a focus on providing continuous care rather than episodic care and using less skilled and less costly providers as part of a multidisciplinary healthcare delivery approach. More critically, organisations support technology-enabled health care reflected in practices and policies regarding the future use of Information and Communications Technology (ICT). At the societal level, the acceptance of a patient-centred and technology-enabled healthcare delivery method is promoted. This promotion involves adapting new interventions (telemedicine) to create environments that reduce defensive medicine [4]. Although the concept of telemedicine is not a recent invention, the global COVID-19 pandemic was a catalyst for the widespread adoption of telemedicine in all areas of healthcare.

While considerable strides have been made regarding telemedicine and its impact on patient and community care, there is a need to proactively (and in some cases retrospectively) ensure patient and system safety, including the security of patient medical data and technologies. As earlier noted, despite the telemedicine processes being implemented quickly considering COVID-19, there is a need to consider if technologies are being utilised safely (e.g., This is very critical, especially when healthcare practitioners handle computing technologies, and while they help provide efficient healthcare, there is always a possibility of either human or software errors to occur. There have not been any studies exploring the application of systemic accident analysis approaches to telemedicine. This chapter explores this gap in addressing the importance of incorporating systems thinking and associated approaches to telemedicine in analysing potential incidents/accidents that may occur using systemic accident analysis (SAA) approaches. The proceeding sections will focus on elaborating three of the most popular SAA approaches applied across different safety-critical industries, including healthcare. Their applications, benefits and limitations will also be discussed.

2. Systemic accident analysis (SAA) approaches

Safety is considered one of the emergent properties of a complex socio-technical system, including the healthcare system [5]. This property is also considered to be very important because of the importance of ensuring the system safety and well-being of patients, professionals, and assets of a health organisation. Different analytical tools have been used to analyse risks and potential hazards that might occur, forming the process of incident/accident analysis [6]. These tools include the popular Root Cause Analysis (RCA) techniques, including Cause and Effect fishbone diagrams, the 5-Whys technique, Change Analysis and Barrier Analysis [7, 8]. However, these linear-based tools have been considered inadequate and unsuitable for analysing complex socio-technical systems [7, 9]. This realisation brought about the development of different systemic accident analysis (SAA) approaches, each based on various safety perspectives, methodologies and theories of accident causation [10, 11]. Some of the most popular examples of this type of approach include AcciMap (Accident Mapping) [12, 13], STAMP/STPA (Systems Theoretic Accident Model and Process) [14, 15], and FRAM (Functional Resonance Accident Model) [16, 17]. These approaches are considered more suitable for analysing incidents that are typically non-linear and involve complex causal relationships stemming from activities at the front line to decisions taken both with and outside health organisations [9]. They have been extensively applied in analysing major incidents within healthcare and other safety-critical domains [7, 18–21]. However, compared to other industries like Aviation, Railway, Nuclear, and Aerospace, the application of these approaches for incident investigation and analysis is still growing in the healthcare industry [7, 22]. These systemic approaches are further elaborated in the proceeding subsections.

2.1 AcciMap mapping (AcciMap)

Svedung and Rasmussen developed this approach as a graphical tool for creating a multi-causal diagram of events and decisions across different socio-technical levels, as shown in **Figure 1** [13, 18, 23–25]. This approach is also based on Rasmussen's theory of accident causation and can be applied either as a standalone method or as a part of a broader Risk Management Framework (RMF) [12, 23]. While there have been different variations of the AcciMap approach, Branford, in her thesis, developed a standardised AcciMap format with a set of guidelines for determining causal/contributing factors, causal relationships between them (linking causal connections within and between socio-technical levels) and formulating safety recommendations [23]. This systemic approach essentially provides the benefit of providing a graphical representation of actions/activities committed at the front end (where clinical practitioners and patients

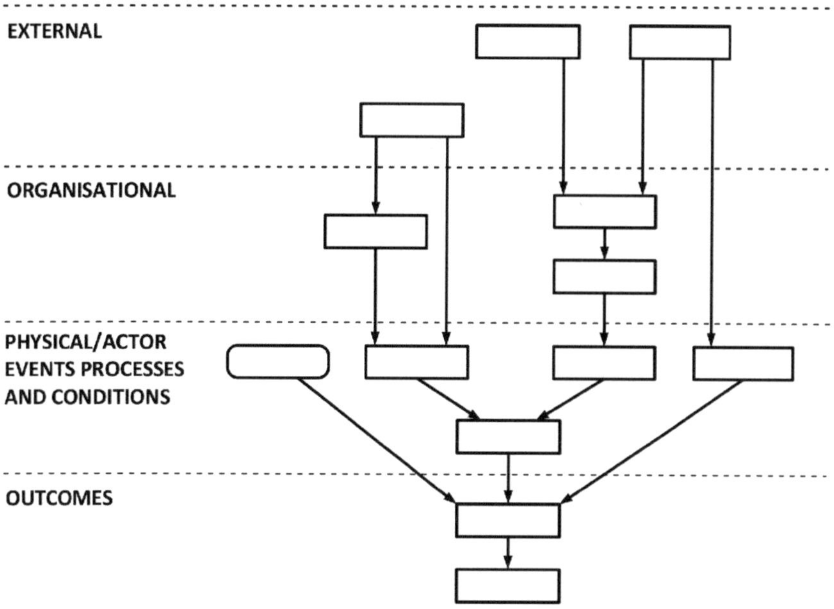

Figure 1.
The standardised AcciMap format [23].

are involved with patients using computing and network technologies) and latent conditions within the health organisation that may have facilitated the events to occur at the front end [21, 26]. Appendix A shows an example application of the AcciMap approach on a medication dosing error relating to a Computerised Order Entry System (CPOE) [21, 27, 28]. The AcciMap approach is based on the safety-I perspective, which essentially involves analysing what went wrong and why it happened so that recommendations can be made to prevent future occurrences.

2.2 Systems theoretic accident modelling process (STAMP)

STAMP is a systemic-based accident approach developed by Leveson (MIT). It is based on systems and control theory regarding safety constraints between various components and determining any disturbances that can potentially affect system safety [9, 15]. As shown in **Figure 2**, the STAMP model consists of a generic socio-

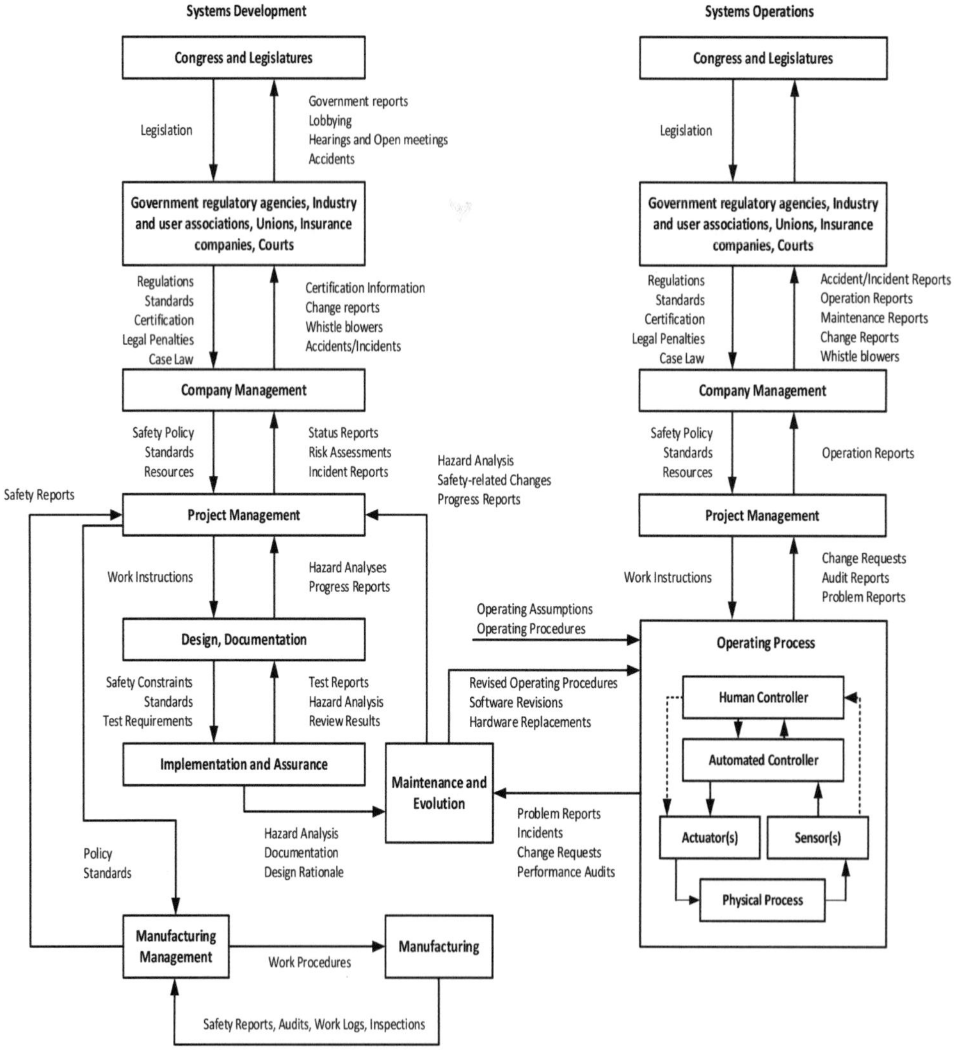

Figure 2.
Generic complex sociotechnical control structure (STAMP Model) [9].

1. Inadequate Enforcements of Constraints (Control Actions)			
	1.1 Unidentified hazards		
	1.2 Inappropriate, ineffective, or missing control actions for identified hazards		
		1.2.1 Design of the control algorithm (process) does not enforce constraints	
			• Flaws in the creation process
			• Process changes without an appropriate change in the control algorithm (asynchronous evolution)
			• Incorrect modification or adaptation
		1.2.2 Process models inconsistent, incomplete or incorrect (lack of linkup)	
			• Flaws in the creation process
			• Flaws in updating process (asynchronous evolution)
			• Time lags and measurement in accuracies not accounted for
		1.2.3 Inadequate coordination among controllers and decision-makers	
2. Inadequate Execution of Control Action			
	2.1 Communication flaw		
	2.2 Inadequate actuator operation		
	2.3 Time lag		
3. Inadequate or Missing Feedback			
	3.1 Not provided in system design		
	3.2 Communication flow		
	3.3 Time lag		
	3.4 Inadequate sensor operation (incorrect or no information provided)		

Table 1.
STAMP's control failure taxonomy of control flaws leading to hazards [14, 15].

technical system safety control structure and a high-level taxonomy of safety constraints for system hazards. An example of the application of the STAMP approach for modelling a high-level control structure relating to the medication dosing error [21, 27] is shown in Appendix B. The STAMP approach also consists of two aspects of analysis; System Theoretic Process Analysis (STPA), which is a STAMP-based hazard analysis used for defining accidents, control structure and system hazards and Causal Analysis using System Theory (CAST) [15, 29]. This model is also based on the traditional safety-I perspective. **Table 1** describes the STAMP's control failure taxonomy of control flaws relating to how they lead to hazards in the system.

STAMP and AcciMap approaches are based on the traditional safety-I perspective, which considers "*safety as the absence of failure or the state in which the fewest number of things go wrong*" [30]. From this safety perspective, there is a shift in blaming the frontline level (actions/activities) to determining existing causal/contributing factors based on decisions at both organisational and external levels.

2.3 Functional resonance accident method (FRAM)

A systemic model was developed by Erik Hollnagel [31], and it's based on "Safety II" perspective that "*identifies and defines systems functions and variability determining*

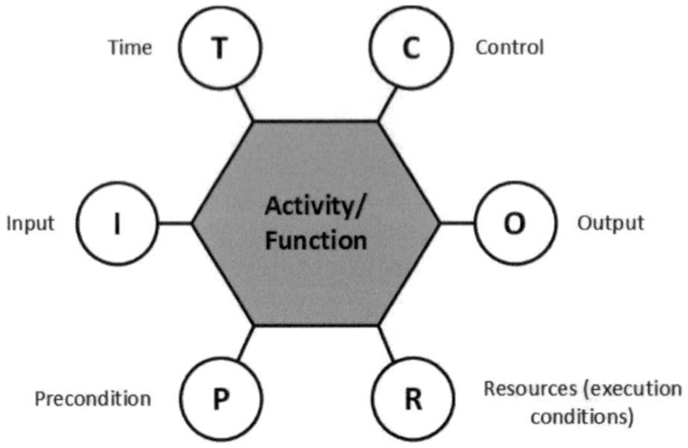

Figure 3.
The FRAM function and associated components [34].

how variability may interact within a system in a manner leading to adverse outcomes" [16]. The development of this model type was motivated by the authors' dissatisfaction with existing approaches like Fault Tree Analysis (FTA) for addressing safety issues [32]. The FRAM model essentially relies on four principles, (a.) Equivalence of successes and failures where they both have the same origin (i.e., performance variability), (b.) Approximate adjustments where people and organisations continually adjust their performances to cope with daily operating challenges, (c.) Emergence, where identifying a sequence of events is considered impossible because many events are seen as emergent rather than a combination of conditions (i.e., latent), and (d.) Functional resonance representing signals coming from unintended interactions of variability (human, organisational and technical behaviours) of multiple signals [33]. A typical representation of the FRAM function is shown in **Figure 3**.

Each FRAM function consists of six [6] components which are briefly highlighted below:

a. Time: Focuses on temporal aspects affecting how the function is accomplished.

b. Input: Triggers the function and can be utilised or transformed to output and linking to upstream functions.

c. Preconditions: Describes conditions of the system that must be carried out before the function is carried out.

d. Control: Focuses on supervision or regulation of a function, including guidelines, procedures, or other functions.

e. Resources (Execution Conditions): Resources, including software, manpower, energy etc., that are utilised or needed by the function.

f. Output: Consists of links to downstream functions, which essentially is the result of the function.

This systemic approach, unlike the last two mentioned (safety-I perspective), is based on the safety-II perspective, which focuses on "*ensuring that as many things as possible go right*" in considering both accidents and outcomes [35]. Based on this safety perspective, human beings are regarded as a resource necessary for system resilience and flexibility, especially when responding to varying conditions [35]. The safety-II view is also considered a proactive approach for anticipating events and allows clinicians' ability to adapt to pressures to be understood. Incident investigations using this perspective (applying the FRAM model) focus on how processes go right and serve as a basis for determining what went wrong [35, 36].

3. Application of SAA approaches

These systemic accident approaches elaborated in the previous section show their analysis methodology and safety perspective on which they are built for accident analysis. While these SAA approaches are graphically oriented in modelling interactions and relationships within a system, AcciMap and STAMP (STPA and CAST) focus mainly on determining weaknesses or loss of control so that safety recommendations can be developed to prevent their reoccurrence (Safety-I). These approaches differ from the FRAM approach, focusing on ensuring that things go right (Safety-II). Their steps regarding how each approach is applied in analysing an incident are highlighted.

3.1 AcciMap analysis process

Regarding applying the AcciMap approach to any incidents to analyse severe outcomes or near-misses, a set of guidelines was formally developed based on Branford's thesis [23, 24] after creating a standardised AcciMap format based on the original AcciMap structure. A graphic template is prepared, which consists of different AcciMap levels and includes the following processes:

a. Identifying the adverse outcome.

b. Determining causal/contributing factors that led to the outcome.

c. Placing contributing factors at the appropriate AcciMap level.

d. Inserting causal links depicting "cause and effect" between causal/contributing factors.

e. Filling any missing gaps in the causal chain where there is missing information.

f. Assessing the causal logic and making sense of any sequence of events.

g. Generating practical and feasible safety recommendations

3.2. STAMP analysis process

There are nine stages involved in applying STAMP, as identified by Leveson [19]. The first eight stages can be carried out, not necessarily in a strict order. When specifically using the Causal Analysis, which is based on STAMP, these stages are summarised as follows:

a. Identify systems and hazards associated with the loss.

b. Identify system safety constraints and requirements relating to the hazard detected.

c. Detail control structures to control the hazard and enforce safety constraints.

d. Determine proximal events that led to the loss.

e. Evaluate the loss at the physical system level.

f. Evaluate the control structure(s) at higher levels.

g. Assess the overall contributors (communication and coordination) to the loss.

h. Determine the changes and dynamics to the control structure and system over time.

i. Develop safety recommendations

3.3 FRAM analysis process

Applying the FRAM method allows positive and negative consequences from work adjustments rather than focusing on causes or contributing factors [37]. There are four processes involved in analysing and developing a FRAM model as follows:

a. Identifying and explaining critical system functions and characterising each one using the six aspects (see **Figure 3**).

b. Distinguish the functions' potential and actual variabilities in multiple model implementations.

c. Determine possible functional resonance based on dependencies with other functions considering their potential/actual variability.

d. Generate safety recommendations that focus on monitoring and influencing the variability. This is achieved either by enhancing the variability leading to desired outcomes or attenuating the variability that can lead to undesired results.

4. Discussion

Each of the SAA approaches addressed in this chapter has been grouped into nine [9] specific categories according to authors Karanikas and Roelen to distinguish them from one another based on their strengths and weaknesses [38]. **Table 2** indicates the SAA approaches strengths (green) and limitations (orange). The subsections will further elaborate on the benefits, demerits and necessity of applying these systemic approaches.

Category	AcciMap	STAMP	FRAM
Graphical Representation	This approach shows causal relationships (links) vertically from the external to the Physical/actor level and can be described in a single diagram. Software tools like Microsoft Vision, Powerpoint and other graphical software can be used to create AcciMap diagrams.	Graphically depicts different system components and processes, including feedback loops between these components to determine any loss of control. A software-specific STAMP visualiser (STAMP workbench) and other graphical tools can be used to create STAMP models.	Graphically creates and analyses different functions and linkages between each function (output to the input of another function), and the accident scene can be represented with a single diagram. Hollnagel developed a FRAM visualiser for this purpose.
		The findings are mostly text-based, with the graphical representation spread across multiple pages.	
Timeline	A proximal sequence of events and influences exists.	Due to the lack of a single graphical representation, there is no clear timeline.	A proximal sequence of events and influences exists. A better timeline can be shown by including time resources and preconditions.
System structure	Rather than system components, this section describes events and actions.	Presents a visual representation of the system hierarchy.	Actions and system components are described.
	There is little information available about the system's structure and boundaries.	Safety constraints define the boundaries of systems.	System boundaries can still be ambiguous.
System component relationships	Only indicates component relationship outputs and how they minimise safety.	Full relationships between components are outlined to determine how dysfunctional interactions lead to decisions/unsafe actions.	Relationships between components are outlined to determine how dysfunctional interactions lead to unsafe system states.
System behaviour	Process details are not provided.	Describes what happened and why unsafe control actions occurred.	Process details are provided.
	Safety objectives are only stated implicitly.	Clearly defines the system and component-level safety objectives at various stages of the analysis.	The objectives for safety are stated explicitly.
Validity	Aims to investigate the dynamic behaviour that exists within a system and how it contributes to accidents	Addresses how the complexity of a system influences the occurrence of accidents.	Clearly states how system variances can contribute to accidents.
Usability	The lack of guidance material makes learning the model a bit more challenging.	Associated guidance materials are substantial	
		Guidance materials can be very complicated to apply, depending on the analysed incident/accident report.	Guidance materials can be relatively challenging to apply, depending on the

Category	AcciMap	STAMP	FRAM
			analysed incident/accident report.
	Lack of jargon language in the analysis	Jargon language is extensively implemented in the analysis.	
System levels	System levels [6] are specified explicitly.	The system levels and columns are specified explicitly.	The system levels are only stated implicitly.
Feedback	No feedback channels	Feedback channels are outlined explicitly	Feedback channels are outlined implicitly.

Table 2.
Strengths and weaknesses of AcciMap, STAMP and FRAM [38].

4.1 Benefits of SAA approaches

Application and comparative studies across different safety-critical industries have highlighted the benefits of applying systemic accident approaches compared to the linear-based approaches in their ability to graphically highlights weaknesses in complex systems and how these systemic issues can create scenarios where actions/activities are committed that could potentially lead to patient harm. The health industry can only continually reap the benefits of using these approaches for incident analysis. Each approach will be further elaborated in specifically examining the benefits of SAA approaches already highlighted in Section 2. For the AcciMap method, its ability to graphically present causal relationships that exist between multiple causal/contributing factors will allow analysts to not only determine causal flows within different socio-technical levels but will also let systemic issues be traced back to the higher levels (organisational and external) and to determine any existing policies and processes that need to be reviewed. The AcciMap approach can be applied by a single analyst but has more benefits when used by a group of analysts (especially having different specialisations within healthcare). The latter process will help foster brainstorming when analysing incidents and producing the initial AcciMap output to the final result after several iterations. Hypotheses can also be drawn based on the AcciMap analysis, and counterfactual reasoning can also be applied when considering sufficient and necessary causes. The STAMP model allows analysts to portray feedback loops between different components within the system graphically. These feedback loops include communication between practitioners and patients (remote connections), as well as with higher bodies and determine any loss of control. Based on the outputs (Appendices A and B), applying both AcciMap and STAMP approaches was used to illustrate and determine systemic factors and any loss of control between system components using a conventional medical scenario. If these approaches were to be applied in a telemedicine scenario, the links between the patient and medical practitioners (communication) would have to be considered. These analyses will also include issues associated with computing technologies applied remotely for communication or administration. When using the AcciMap method, these aspects can be analysed at the physical/actor level to determine if there was any miscommunication between staff and patient, defects in technology used, and what conditions precipitated it. The STAMP model can also be applied in a telemedical scenario when feedback loops can be analysed to determine any loss of control when looking into issues regarding remote administration and communication (or lack of) between patients and staff. The FRAM model can also be applied in a telemedical situation. However, compared to conventional medicine, the difference is that aspects regarding how technology is "remotely" implemented in communicating and providing patient care will need to be analysed if there are any accidents, near-misses or loss of control. Other aspects can also include patient or medical staff misapplication and accessibility of technology.

4.2 Demerits of SAA approaches

It is also important that while there are benefits to applying systemic approaches, the demerits must also be highlighted. Major drawbacks of using systemic models for incident analysis as applied to telemedicine are resources required in terms of personnel, time, and knowledge needed to apply them effectively. Depending on the approach used, it can take considerable time and effort to understand the causation theory and methodology behind each approach and to apply them to analyse any major incident(s) in healthcare. Also, about this point, it is very important to take into consideration when it comes to each systemic approach's validity, reliability and usability in producing results that will allow effective safety recommendations to be formulated (retrospectively) and that these safety measures can then be tracked and assessed to ensure that any weaknesses detected will not occur again. While each approach can be applied individually, as each analytical iteration can be reviewed, it is usually recommended that multiple users (team-based) apply the approach to the same incident. This step will allow brainstorming and discussions to produce the final outcome. Health organisations will also require training of staff associated with risk management and computing technology in applying different systemic approaches, which could also take a considerable amount of time. These points highlight why Root Cause Analysis (RCA) techniques are still being used because they do not require as much time in terms of training and application. Still, as stated earlier in this chapter, their underlying methodologies are not considered suitable for analysing complex systems. However, this limitation is somewhat circumvented when using software-based modelling tools based on some systemic approaches. For instance, there are a FRAM visualiser and STAMP Workbench applications for FRAM and STAMP/STPA analyses, respectively. Microsoft Visio application or other graphic tools can construct AcciMap outputs during analysis.

4.3 The Necessity of SAA approaches

Considering the benefits and demerits discussed in previous subsections, it stands to reason that health organisations will need to weigh these benefits versus the limitations of applying these approaches for incident analysis relating to telemedicine. Based on previous studies comparing systemic approaches with other linear-based and systemic-based models [7, 11, 21], there is a clear conclusion that applying the systems thinking paradigm is the way forward in analysing, understanding, and improving system safety relating to telemedicine. This point also encompasses processes that are involved when it comes to telemedicine as far as healthcare professionals and patients are concerned. It is very important to acknowledge the general limitations of these approaches mentioned and understand that there are tangible benefits depending on which systemic approach is implemented. While there have been studies investigating how the "*research-practice gap*" as coined by Underwood and Waterson [39], can be reduced in terms of applying these approaches in healthcare, there is still a need for providing awareness to clinical safety and risk managers. Aside from the need to improve system safety by ensuring that whatever safety recommendations or mitigating processes are set in place relating to telemedicine processes, there is also a need to protect patient medical data from hacking and other breaches. This issue of patient data being hacked relates to cyber security, especially when the connection is over an unencrypted or public network [40]. The STAMP model can also be applied to analyse this type of security-related incident by implementing an STPA analysis specifically for cyber security analysis called STPA-SafeSec (System-Theoretic Process Analysis for Safety and Security) [41–43]. The authors added that STPA could be applied to analyse system safety and security and systems regarding emerging properties. Security analysis using STPA-Sec serves as a means of ensuring the safety of patient medical data for telemedicine, according to Young and Leveson. They also indicated that safety and security must be addressed collectively [41, 42].

5. Conclusions

There is a need to consider the importance of incident analysis relating to telemedicine to improve practices/processes and ultimately improve safety and security relating to patients, medical data, health professionals and health organisations. Applying systems thinking by utilising systemic approaches will help to graphically model interactions in complex socio-technical systems and detect weaknesses by examining causal/contributing factors, causal relationships, and any communication and feedback loops within the system. However, applying these approaches requires considerable resources regarding awareness, training, and proper application of guidelines to realise their necessary benefits and improve the process of telemedicine.

Acknowledgements

There is no funding information relating to the work of this chapter.

Conflict of interest

There are no conflicts of interest relating to the contributions for this chapter from the authors.

Appendix A: AcciMap Analysis of the Medication Dosing Error related to the CPOE system

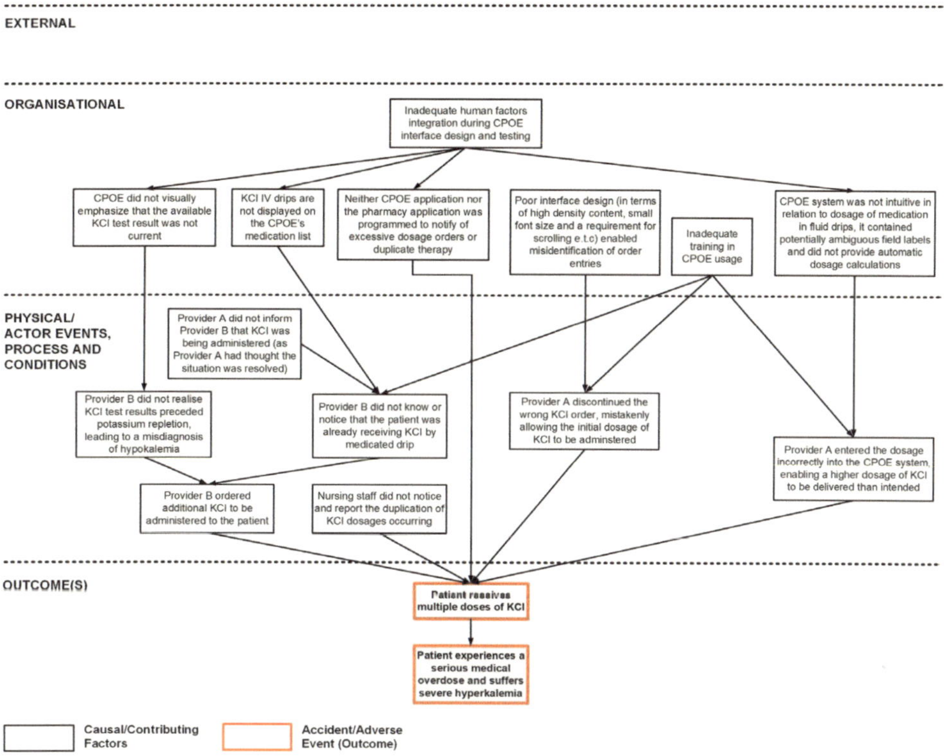

Appendix B: The STAMP Control Structure of the CPOE Medication Error Case Study

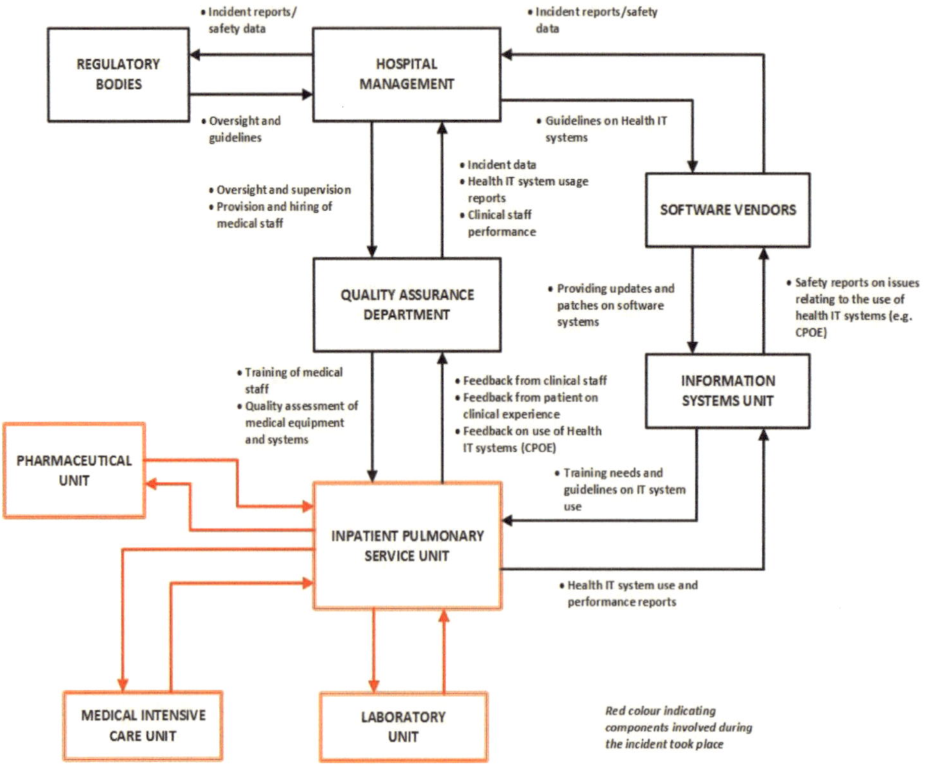

Author details

Oseghale Igene[1*] and Aimee Ferguson[2]

1 University of Glasgow, Glasgow, United Kingdom

2 University of Strathclyde, Glasgow, United Kingdom

*Address all correspondence to: oseigene@hotmail.com

References

[1] Perednia DA, Allen A. Telemedicine technology and clinical applications. Journal of the American Medical Association. 1995;**273**(6):483-488

[2] Hjelm NM. Benefits and drawbacks of telemedicine. Journal of Telemedicine and Telecare. 2005;**11**(2):60-70

[3] Craig J, Petterson V. Introduction to the Practice of Telemedicine. 2016;**11**(1): 3-9. DOI: 101177/1357633X0501100102

[4] Heinzelmann PJ, Lugn NE, Kvedar JC. Telemedicine in the future. Journal of Telemedicine and Telecare. 2005;**11**(8):384-390

[5] Leveson NG. Rasmussen's legacy: A paradigm change in engineering for safety. Applied Ergonomics. 2017;**59**:581-591

[6] Johnson CW. An introduction to Root Cause Analysis in healthcare. 2004. p. 1–47. Available from: http://www.dcs.gla.ac.uk/~johnson/papers/Pascale_book/incident_analysis.PDF

[7] Canham A, Thomas Jun G, Waterson PE, Khalid S. Integrating systemic accident analysis into patient safety incident investigation practices. Applied Ergonomics. 2018;**72**:1-9

[8] Dixon K, Waterson PE, Barnes J. A comparison of three systemic accident analysis methods using 46 SPAD (Signals passed at danger) incidents. In: Advances in Intelligent Systems and Computing. Los Angeles, USA: Springer Verlag; 2018. pp. 1097-1108

[9] Leveson NG. Applying systems thinking to analyse and learn from events. Safety Science. 2011;**49**(1):55-64

[10] Underwood P., Waterson PE. Accident analysis models and methods: Guidance for safety professionals. 2013

[11] Underwood P, Waterson P. A critical review of the stamp, fram and accimap systemic accident analysis models. In: Advances in Human Aspects of Road and Rail Transportation. 2012

[12] Rasmussen J, Svedung I. Proactive risk management in a dynamic society. In: Swedish Rescue Services Agency. Karlstad, Sweden: Risk and Environmental Department; 2000. pp. 1-160. Available from: http://rib.msb.se/Filer/pdf%5C16252.pdf

[13] Svedung I, Rasmussen J. Graphic representation of accident scenarios: Mapping system structure and the causation of accidents. Safety Science. 2002;**40**(5):397-417

[14] Leveson NG. System safety engineering: Back to the future. Aeronautics and Astronautics Massachusetts Institute of Technology; Cambridge. 2002. p. 1–320. Available from: http://sunnyday.mit.edu/book2.pdf

[15] Leveson NG. A new accident model for engineering safer systems. Safety Science. 2004;**42**(4):237-270

[16] Hollnagel E. FRAM, the Functional Resonance Analysis Method: Modelling Complex Socio-Technical Systems. Farnham, Surrey, UK: Ashgate Publishing Ltd; 2012

[17] Hollnagel E. An application of Functional Resonance Analysis Method (FRAM) to Risk Assessment of Organisational Change. Stockholm: Strålskyddsnämnden (SSN). 2013

[18] Salmon PM, Cornelissen M, Trotter MJ. Systems-based accident analysis methods: A comparison of

Accimap, HFACS, and STAMP. Elsevier Ltd. 2012;**50**(4):1158-1170

[19] Underwood P, Waterson PE. Systems thinking, the Swiss Cheese Model and accident analysis: A comparative systemic analysis of the Grayrigg train derailment using the ATSB, AcciMap and STAMP models. Accident; Analysis and Prevention. 2014;**68**:75-94

[20] Kee D, Jun GT, Waterson P, Haslam R. A systemic analysis of South Korea Sewol ferry accident – Striking a balance between learning and accountability. Applied Ergonomics. Mar 2017;**1**(59):504-516

[21] Igene OO, Johnson C. Analysis of medication dosing error related to computerised provider order entry system: A comparison of ECF, HFACS, STAMP and AcciMap approaches. Health Informatics Journal. 2019;**26**(2): 1017-1042

[22] Igene OO, Johnson C. To computerised provider order entry system: A comparison of ECF, HFACS, STAMP and AcciMap approaches. Health Informatics Journal. 2020;**26**(2): 1017-1042

[23] Branford K. An Investigation into the Validity and Reliability of the AcciMap Approach. Australia: The Australian National University; 2007

[24] Branford K, Naikar N, Hopkins A. Guidelines for AcciMap analysis. In: Hopkins A, editor. Learn from High Reliab Organ Sydney CCH. 2009. pp. 193-212

[25] Lee S, Moh YB, Tabibzadeh M, Meshkati N. Applying the AcciMap methodology to investigate the tragic Sewol Ferry accident in South Korea. Applied Ergonomics. 2017;**59**:517-525

[26] Igene OO, Johnson CW, Long J. An evaluation of the formalised AcciMap approach for accident analysis in healthcare. Cognition, Technology & Work. 2021:1-21

[27] Horsky J, Kuperman GJ, Patel VL. Comprehensive analysis of a medication dosing error related to CPOE. Journal of the American Medical Informatics Association. 2005;**12**(4): 377-382

[28] Igene OO, Johnson CW. Comparing HFACS and AcciMaps in a health informatics case study - The analysis of a medication dosing error. In: Safety and Reliability - Safe Societies in a Changing World. ESREL 2018: Proceedings of the 28th International European Safety and Reliability Conference; 2018. pp. 3-10

[29] Leveson N, Daouk M, Dulac N, Marais K. Applying STAMP in accident analysis. NASA Conference. 2003: 177-198. Available from: https://ntrs.nasa.gov/api/citations/20030111708/downloads/20030111708.pdf

[30] Smaggus A. Safety-I, Safety-II and Burnout: How Complexity Science Can Help Clinician Wellness. Vol. 28. BMJ Quality and Safety. BMJ Publishing Group; 2019. pp. 667-671

[31] Hollnagel E. Barriers and Accident Prevention. London, Aldershot, UK: Ashgate; 2004

[32] Grant E, Salmon PM, Stevens NJ, Goode N, Read GJ. Back to the Future: What do Accident Causation Models tell us About Accident Prediction? Vol. 104. Safety Science. Elsevier B.V; 2018. pp. 99-109

[33] Riccardo P, Gianluca DP, Giulio DG, Francesco C. FRAM for Systemic

accident analysis: A matrix representation of functional resonance. International Journal of Reliability, Quality and Safety Engineering. 2018 Feb;**25**(1):1, 1-29

[34] Flin R, Winter J, Cakil Sarac MR. Human factors in patient safety: Review of topics and tools. World Health. 2009;**2**

[35] Hollnagel E, Wears R, Braithwaite J. From safety-i to safety-II: A white paper from safety-I to safety-II: A white paper. In: Safety-II: A White Paper From Safety-I to Safety-II: A White. 2015: 1-43. DOI: 10.13140/RG.2.1.4051. 5282.o

[36] Finkel M. On Flexibility: Recovery from Technological and Doctrinal Surprise on the Battlefield. Stanford, CA: Stanford University Press; 2011

[37] Hollnagel E, Hounsgaard J, Colligan L. FRAM-the Functional Resonance Analysis Method-a Handbook for the Practical Use of the Method. 2014. p. 75

[38] Karanikas N, Roelen A. The Concept Towards a Standard Safety Model (STASAM). MATEC Web Conf; 2019

[39] Underwood P, Waterson PE. Systemic accident analysis: Examining the gap between research and practice. Accident; Analysis and Prevention. 2013; **1**(55):154-164

[40] Haleem A, Javaid M, Singh RP, Suman R. Telemedicine for healthcare: Capabilities, features, barriers, and applications. Sensors International. 2021; **1**(2):100117

[41] Young W, Leveson N. Systems thinking for safety and security. Proceedings of the 29th Annual Computer Security Applications Conference. 2013

[42] Young W, Leveson NG. An integrated approach to safety and security based on systems theory. Communications of the ACM. 2014;**57**(2):31-35

[43] Friedberg I, McLaughlin K, Smith P, Laverty D, Sezer S. STPA-SafeSec: Safety and security analysis for cyber-physical systems. Journal of Information Security and Applications. 2017;**34**:183-196

Chapter 9

Addressing Pain Points: Thinking outside the Telehealth Box

Lua Perimal-Lewis, Patricia A.H. Williams, Ginger Mudd and Gihan Gunasekara

Abstract

In this chapter, we present the synthesis of six pain points relating to Australia's hospital congestion which is under crisis. The COVID-19 pandemic forced health services to respond rapidly to maintain continuity of care through telehealth. Some of these strategies were anticipated to be short-term arrangements, implemented quickly, and haphazardly deployed. While the health emergency accelerated the adoption of telehealth and models of remote care, this implementation was reactive. It is evident that our hospital systems continue to grapple with the issues of an aging population, expanding demand for mental health services, and escalating costs and too few resources. A shift in philosophy to address these and other recurring pain points presents opportunities to embrace virtual care beyond current implementations of telehealth.

Keywords: telehealth, virtual care, healthcare pain point, hospital congestion, pandemic

1. Introduction

It was a leisurely Sunday afternoon in a small country town with children playing happily until a freak accident on the playground "hamster wheel." A possible fractured finger and a trip to the Emergency Department (ED). Calling ahead to notify the ED of our arrival, the nurse replied, *"Good timing, I was about to head off!"*. The rural ED with a quaint cottage like frontage (complete with doorbell) revealed an empty waiting room. The nurse greeted us and returned with a pile of paper-based forms. Apparently, the doctor on-call would arrive shortly. She joked upon seeing a 30-year-old man, *"I was expecting to see a four-year-old!"*. She confirmed a fracture but advised that she is not able to treat the injury until they could find the radiologist. Since there were no other patients in the waiting room, she went home to feed her 2-year-old. The radiologist arrived after 30 minutes. Within minutes the ED became busy with other presentations; (A) an older patient recently discharged from hospital arrived by an ambulance, (B) a worried young father holding a baby with gastro, (C) a young man with a drug overdose and mental health condition, and (D) another older patient with an allergic reaction to his eyes after tending to the weeds in his garden. The doctor returned to an (E) overcrowded ED but was calm and collected and

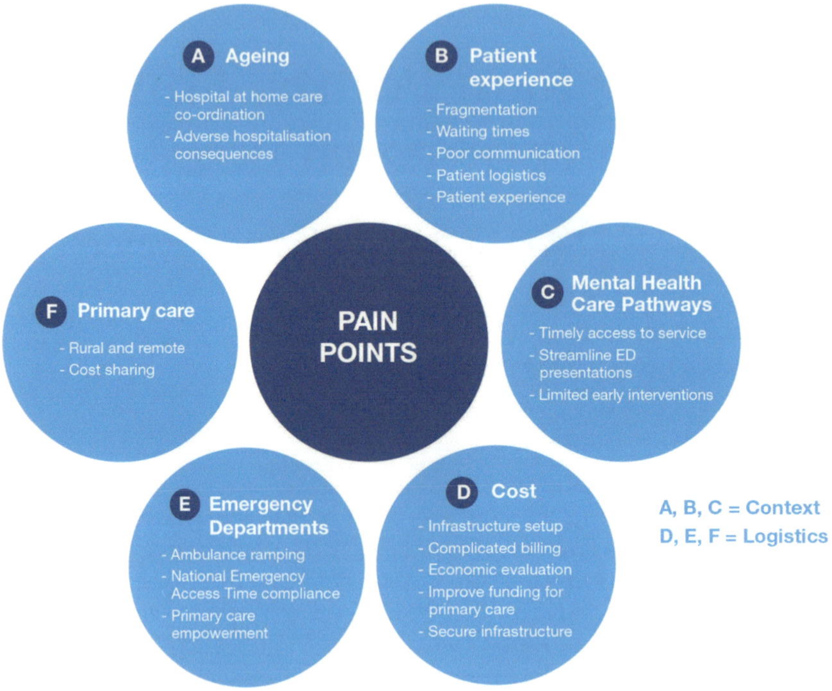

Figure 1.
Australia's recurring healthcare challenges [1, 2].

did a stellar job in attending to all the patients. Despite the chaos, the lack of privacy, the uncertainty, and the frustration of waiting, all the patients were cared for with the limited resources.

As for the fractured finger, the doctor communicated via mobile phone with consultants at a metro hospital, located hundreds of kilometeres away. The X-ray was sent via WhatsApp to the senior consultant and to us (F). Eventually, we left with a taped splint and painkillers.

This real ED experience highlights the issues and pain points (see **Figure 1**) that clinicians at acute care setting have to deal with on a daily basis, and at scale for busy metropolitan hospitals. These recurring issues impact patients, healthcare providers, and the government. Worldwide, such pain points are worsening demanding that hospital administrators and policymakers understand the complexity of these multilevel interactions and look outside of the acute care settings to improve patient outcomes.

This chapter discusses how telehealth and the evolution to virtual care can begin to address the major pain points faced by overburdened hospitals as well as enhance the patient experience.

2. The evolution of telehealth to virtual care?

Virtual care is a broad term for all the digital tools and real-time communication, to enable healthcare providers to remotely work together with the patient [1]. In Australia, like many countries, health services are stretched and faced with an increasing burden from an aging population, rising costs, and increasing demand

(**Figure 1**). Telehealth was vastly underutilized prior to the COVID-19 pandemic. The global response prompted a broad and reactive adoption of telehealth. In Australia, there was a 35% increase in use over only a 2-month period in early 2020 [3]. Greater increases were seen worldwide. In addition, research has shown that consumer acceptance of telehealth has been high and a predominantly positive experience [4].

While telehealth can be defined as the use of telecommunication techniques for the purpose of providing telemedicine, medical education and health education over distance [5, 6], and telemedicine uses advanced technologies [5, 7], virtual care refers to the delivery of patient-centered, cost-effective, and timely clinical care from a distance such as real-time video interaction and online exchange of information between a patient and their doctor and/or clinical team [8]. A wide perspective is needed to rethink delivery of healthcare that ensures continuity of care across multiple providers that can be delivered outside of acute care hospital environments.

As technology, in particular home and remote monitoring devices, evolve, the opportunity to support remote care using technology has increased. In Australia, this is now coined as virtual care to characterize a more complete experience for the patient, rather than telehealth consultation which can be anything from a 5-minute telephone call to a video consultation. It is unfortunate that because of the rapid deployment during COVID-19, the medical interaction was often second to the management and inexperience with the technology. As patients and clinicians have become more familiar with the technology, there is an opportunity to support consultations with home monitoring devices.

The following sections briefly discuss these pain points by giving select evidence where the underlying solution is outside of the acute care settings.

2.1 Aging

Most older patients presenting at acute care settings have multiple chronic conditions and a higher risk of hospital readmission for complications attributed to a different primary condition to the indexed admission [9]. Therefore, recently discharged older patients with chronic health conditions require a well-coordinated solution at home. Simulating a hospital environment, these patients can be effectively managed at home using remote patient monitoring devices or wearables that continuously monitor the patient's condition by tracking vital signs and medication compliance. The data collected is sent to the clinicians allowing them to monitor, identify symptoms, and intervene early. Reducing hospitalization will benefit older patients who are more likely to be affected by adverse drug events [10] and hospital acquired infections which prolong Length of Stay. The implementation and sustainability of virtual care for older adults is contingent on better integration of technology into their lives as well as healthcare providers [11]. Although still in its early stages, experience shows that technologies used in hospital at home are safe and acceptable to both patients and clinicians, as well as it reduces the ongoing resource tension at acute care settings [12].

2.2 Patient experience

Healthcare organizations are striving to provide patient-centered care, yet a long way from addressing the most prevalent patient pain points such as care fragmentation, long waiting times, poor doctor-patient communication, and poor logistics in hospitals, all of which contribute to compromised care and services that are not personalized to the individual [13]. Analysis of patient satisfaction has been part of healthcare service review for a number of years; however, there is a move from satisfaction to patient experience which is a proxy for one of the six indicators of quality healthcare in the US [14]. The "young father and the baby with gastro" is a classic example of care fragmentation. It was evident when the ED doctor attended to this patient, that the baby has other chronic illness managed by other services. The patient has navigated the health system by moving from one health service to another, and there was lack of communication between the various service providers. Communication is a key factor in measuring patient experience [15, 16]. Fragmentation across continuum of care is common because of the very nature of a patient's journey through disparate systems, availability of medical data, and lack of real-time data sharing. It is the development of secure and scalable digital infrastructure that is the foundation to facilitate a coherent patient journey by moving to an increasingly connected and integrated healthcare system.

2.3 Mental healthcare

Another pain point for the government is the management of mental health patients who tend to have longer wait times in ED, often requiring more time for stabilization and/or to complete investigations and are more likely to present after hours, suggesting the need for community-based services [17]. Reconceptualizing mental health service delivery requires organizations to traverse beyond telehealth; mental health professionals need to embrace smartphone-based digital technology such as Ecological Momentary Assessment (EMA) for continuous monitoring and early intervention outside of acute care, so on demand care can be offered before an adverse event. The "young man with drug overdose and mental health issues" was a regular visitor and could have been better managed outside of ED using EMA. Embracing digital health technology would enable service providers to transition care outside of health facilities by means of continuous digital touchpoints enabling irregularities in behaviors identified in real time, alerting a crisis. A well-implemented virtual care platform can enable continuous data collection from active monitoring and passive sensor data to deliver personalized and timely intervention.

2.4 Costs

The Australian healthcare funding model is complex in nature, funded by all levels of government—federal, state, territory, and local. Virtual care service provision, enabling care outside of acute care settings, will drive innovation in funding as demonstrated during COVID-19, but more is needed. The cost savings gained by keeping patients out of hospitals could be diverted for the setup of virtual care infrastructure, improving primary care funding and extending Medicare supported service provision by allied health professionals. The "patient presenting with allergic reaction to his eyes" could be better managed at a primary care health facility, which was nonexistent in the small country town. Innovative funding model to find synergies on how the government fund primary care will be the driving factor to improve poor health outcomes in rural and remote communities, with less reliance on larger urban centeres. The ED doctor who had to communicate with consultants at a metro hospital is a case in point. In addition, it is vital that all communication regarding a patient is through a secure platform rather than via WhatsApp which poses unprecedented data sharing noncompliance risk. Prioritizing funding to finance secure platforms with the agility of WhatsApp that ensures confidentiality, privacy of patient, and clinical data should dominate federal healthcare funding conversation.

2.5 Emergency department

Waiting times is a key issue in Eds, with hospitals under pressure to meet National Emergency Access Target targets [18]. Enabling virtual care assessment, management of low acuity patients, and devising innovative ways to empower primary care physicians to keep patients out of hospital would reduce ED presentations, waiting times, and ambulance ramping. Investment into processes and identifying care pathways that can triage patients that do not need hospitalization such as the vast majority of psychiatric patients by offering appropriate interventions and connection to community/primary care would naturally reduce the pressure on ED and would allow emergency resources to be better utilized for more serious cases.

2.6 Primary care

Access to health services remains a problem for residents of isolated settlements [19]. Virtual care is a vital component to addressing this issue. While "telehealth" and "telemedicine" have been widely used in Australia over the past decade as a means of overcoming problems of access to healthcare and the shortage of health professionals in rural and remote areas [20]; in many cases, telemedicine and telehealth are used to augment other service delivery models [19]. There is a need to ensure a comprehensive range of well-coordinated primary healthcare and specialist services are accessible locally and virtual care should be part of this solution, particularly as the prevalence of chronic disease grows with the aging of Australia's rural and remote population [19]. A well-coordinated, technology-enabled acute to primary and specialist care pathways will streamline the process of follow-ups post discharge.

3. Discussion

Sustainable and effective virtual care provision, with telehealth as part of this, is the way forward for healthcare in Australia. Creating a virtual care environment

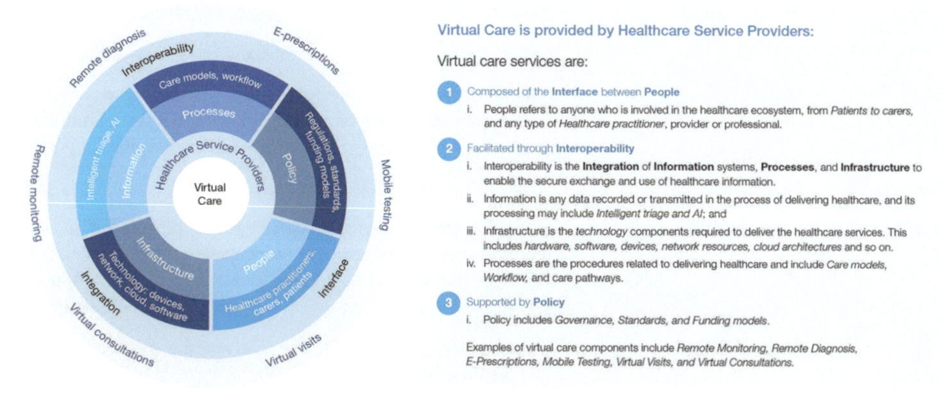

Figure 2.
Virtual care components [1, 2].

means looking at the pain points more broadly from the perspective of how a care team rather than acute services can address the challenges. These solutions must be cognizant of the patient and healthcare provider user experience, fit into clinical workflows and care processes, and supported by the integration of technologies with information systems underpinned by seamless communication. They must also be interoperable, scalable, and secure (**Figure 2**).

These components allow the collation of technologies to generate accessing, sharing, coordinating operations, and security capabilities. These capabilities facilitate the interface between people and integration of information with care processes.

In addition to the virtual care components, there are several actions needed to support the ongoing and increased adoption of virtual care and telehealth in Australia and across the world. Funding and reimbursement for services both for consumers and providers, and investment in infrastructure to support service delivery are issues that need attention given that 7 million people (28% of the population) live in rural

Device category	Device types	Health application
Medical devices	Skin patch sensors	Multi-electrode bioelectronics technology is used for physiological sign monitoring, e.g. pulse, temperature, as well as electrocardiogram (ECG) and electroencephalogram (EEG) readings together with physical activity and sleep patterns. Ultrasound technology is used for cardiac monitoring and diagnosis monitoring blood flow through blood vessels.
	Skin patch for therapeutics	Used for delivery of chemotherapy into melanoma tumors.
	Heart rate monitors	Uses optical (wrist, arm bands or in-ear) or electrical (chest straps) technology.
	Blood pressure monitors	Ambulatory BP monitoring and home BP monitoring devices using finger, wrist, and arm cuff technology, often with Bluetooth communications.
	Smart contact lens	Uses IoT technology to monitor for diabetes, glaucoma, and cataracts.
Accessories	Hearing aids	AI enhanced hearing aids can track blood pressure, notify loved ones in the event of a fall, track activity, and potentially predict early signs of dementia.
	Smartwatches	Fitness tracking, sleep monitoring, and ECG heart reading.
	Fitness trackers	Pedometer (step count), heart rate, and sleep monitoring
	Smart glasses	For use by the partially sighted or blind, connecting glasses to a sighted person. Connecting clinical care specialists in acute care scenarios to one another for instance during operations.
Fashion	Smart jewelery	Step tracking, heart rate, and sleep monitoring
E-textiles	Smart clothing	IoT-based textiles integrated with electronic devices for monitoring heart rate, respiration rates, sleep, and temperature. Examples include smart socks can detect foot ulcer development and smart swimsuits that alert when sunscreen should be applied.
	Smart shoes	Tracking steps, speed, stride rate, foot landing, ground contact, and monitor fatigue on feet.

Table 1.
Examples of the types of devices that have monitoring and diagnostic functions and their application.

and remote areas in Australia [21]. Another challenge is the integration of virtual care services into routine care and clinical workflows. In Australia, many telehealth consultations were via the telephone only and did not result in optimal healthcare delivery [22]. This in turn also requires a competent workforce to utilize virtual care and new or adopted models of care. As virtual care is dependent of the use technology, there is a need to invest in support structures and infrastructure which includes an ecosystem that supports wearable technology.

Wearable technology can be worn on the body or implanted. They collect data directly from the person and communicate it with other connected devices such as a smartphone or computer, using Bluetooth or the Internet. Digital natives are likely to use these wearable devices without much hesitation, but digital immigrants may need some persuasion. However, a recent study found that older adults, especially those who are familiar with smartphones, are interested in using wearable devices and joining online health community enabling aging in place [23]. **Table 1** lists examples of the types of devices that have monitoring and diagnostic functions and their application.

Like aging in place philosophy, a shift to deliver care in place could see select emergency care generally offered in the ED are taken to patients triaged suitable to receive such care. Patients could be assessed in the comfort of their environment by paramedics connected to emergency physicians located at the hospital through a secure video link. Once stabilized, patients could be left with a remote monitoring device which will continue to send life feed to the clinicians at the hospital who can intervene in an event of health deterioration. The remote monitoring and care can continue until the patient can be safely discharged to primary care services in the community, preventing repeat hospital visits or admission soon after discharge like the older patient who presented at the ED described in the scenario above. The availability of data on the electronic consultation as well as the availability of remote monitoring data can facilitate better informed clinical decision-making based on the trend of the collected data. Such data availability is almost nonexistent in the traditional modality. For an emergency physician who is normally exposed to a chaotic ED environment, a virtual care modality where that care is delivered virtually from the comfort of their home would aid better judgment, thus improving patient outcome and contributing to a less stressed workforce.

4. Conclusions

In the ED presentations described here, there are many opportunities which can be explored using virtual care that could have prevented almost all of these presentations. There is no framework for how to move forward with virtual care in a comprehensive manner in Australia [24, 25]. Without an inclusive and all-encompassing framework for virtual care adoption, the facets it comprises, its challenges and what benefits it can realize, it is not possible to innovate and devise solutions to address these patient and government pain points.

It is the combination of people, monitoring and communication technology, process, infrastructure, information, and policy that form the basis for the future for virtual care solutions to become part of the common practice. Ultimately, it is the benefits for the patient, healthcare providers, and healthcare system that virtual care can deliver that will drive the medium- and long-term adoption. Virtual care has the potential to reform healthcare, providing patient-centered care with more convenience, less costs, and greater productivity.

On a national basis, governments need to devise clear roadmaps for digital health innovation in virtual care to reduce costs and improve accessibility and health outcomes, while solving the acute care sector pain points. Funding, leadership, and policy are key success factors that will strengthen its adoption to realize improvements in patient outcomes. For rural and remote communities in particular, research into the efficacy of remote monitoring and wearable device collected data to support patient-centered healthcare decision-making and patient outcomes will contribute to the introduction of outcomes-based funding models.

From an industry perspective, upskilling the workforce to deliver virtual care services as well as new integrated models of care will help meet the increasing demand for services. Future opportunities using augmented and virtual reality open up new avenues for education of the healthcare workforce in innovative ways.

Ultimately, awareness of virtual care by patients and consumers increased due to COVID-19. The rapid adoption of the technology, arguably not well thought out in the rush, needs to be reassessed to focus on the improvement and reliability and transparency, so that the focus can be on the clinical iteration and patient outcomes rather than the technology used to achieve the communication.

A bold vision needs to emerge for an information and technology enabled healthcare system, where care is virtualized and enabled where it is needed, rather than where it is available. It is a system where clinicians and patients can communicate effectively and one in which clinical process is centered around the needs of the patient. Most importantly, it is an environment in which the patient is better engaged and supported in their journey to wellness. Concerted efforts are needed to systematically, rigorously test and evaluate the impact of various modality of care virtualization to address healthcare pain points.

Acknowledgements

Cisco Systems Australia is acknowledged for their kind finding contribution to the research project in virtual care.

Conflict of interest

The authors declare no conflict of interest.

Author details

Lua Perimal-Lewis*, Patricia A.H. Williams, Ginger Mudd and Gihan Gunasekara
Cisco-Flinders Digital Health Design Lab, Flinders University of South Australia, Adelaide, Australia

*Address all correspondence to: lua.perimal-lewis@flinders.edu.au

References

[1] Williams PAH, et al. Reimagining a Better Healthcare System through Virtual Care. 2020. Available at: https://www.cisco.com/c/dam/en_us/solutions/industries/resources/healthcare/reimagining-better-healthcare-system-through-virtual-care.pdf. [Accessed: 9 November 2022]

[2] Perimal-lewis L, et al. Virtual Care: The Future for Telehealth. IOS Press; 2021:106-113

[3] Thomas EE et al. Building on the momentum: Sustaining telehealth beyond COVID-19. Journal of Telemedicine and Telecare. 2022;**28**(4):301-308

[4] Manski-nankervis J-A et al. Primary care consumers' experiences and opinions of a telehealth consultation delivered via video during the covid-19 pandemic. Australian Journal of Primary Health. 2022;**28**(3):224-231

[5] Australian Institute of Health and Welfare. Australia's Health 2020 Data Insights. Canberra: Australian Institute of Health and Welfare; 2020

[6] International Organization for Standardization [ISO]. ISO/TR 14639-1 Health Informatics - Capacity-based ehealth Architecture Roadmap. ISO; 2012

[7] International Organization for Standardization [ISO]. ISO/TR 16056 Health Informatics - Interoperability of Telehealth Systems and Networks, Interoperability of Tele-learning Systems. ISO; 2004

[8] Schwamm LH, Erskine A, Licurse A. A digital embrace to blunt the curve of covid19 pandemic. NPJ Digital Medicine. 2020;**3**(1):64

[9] Westley-wise V et al. Patterns of morbidity and multimorbidity associated with early and late readmissions in an australian regional health service. Chronic Illness. 2022;**2022**:1742

[10] Paradissis C et al. The type and incidence of adverse drug events in ageing medical inpatients and their effect on length of hospital stay. Journal of Pharmacy Practice and Research. 2017;**47**(5):347-354

[11] Watt JA et al. Barriers and facilitators to virtual care in a geriatric medicine clinic: A semi-structured interview study of patient, caregiver and healthcare provider perspectives. Age and Ageing. 2022;**51**(1):Afab218

[12] Conley J et al. Technology-enabled hospital at home: Innovation for acute care at home. Nejm Catalyst Innovations in Care Delivery. 2022;**3**:Catalysis 21.0402

[13] Radenkovic B. et al. Progressing the patient experience in iot connected healthcare, H. Series, editor. 2018

[14] Golda N et al. Analysis of the patient experience measure. Journal of American Academy Dermatology. 2018;**78**(4):645-651

[15] Street RL et al. How does communication heal? Pathways linking clinician-patient communication to health outcomes. Patient Education Counselling. 2009;**74**(3):295-301

[16] Street R. How clinician-patient communication contributes to health improvement: Modeling pathways from talk to outcome. Patient Education Counselling. 2013;**92**(3):286-291

[17] Shafiei T, Gaynor N, Farrell G. The characteristics, management and

outcomes of people identified with Mental Health issues in an Emergency Department, Melbourne, Australia. Journal of Psychiatric and Mental Health Nursing. 2011;**18**(1):9

[18] Perimal-Lewis L. et al. The relationship between in-hospital location and outcomes of care in patients of a large general medical service. Internal Medicine Journal. 2013;**43**(6):712-716

[19] Kuipers W. et al. Primary health care delivery models in rural and remote australia—A systematic review. 2010

[20] Carey TA et al. What is the overall impact or effectiveness of visiting primary health care services in rural and remote communities in high-income countries? A systematic review. BMC Health Services Research. 2018;**18**(1):476

[21] Australian Institute of Health and Welfare, Rural and Remote Health. Australian Institute of Health and Welfare: Canberra. 2022

[22] Rush LL et al. Videoconference compared to telephone in healthcare delivery: A systematic review. International Journal of Medical Information. 2018;**118**:44-53

[23] Wang J et al. Mobile and connected health technology needs for older adults aging in place: Cross-sectional survey study. JMIR Aging. 2019;**2**:E13864

[24] Shaw J et al. Virtual care policy recommendations for patient-centred primary care: Findings of a consensus policy dialogue using a nominal group technique. Journal of Telemedicne Telecare. 2018;**24**(9):608-615

[25] Waller M, Stotler C. Telemedicine: A primer. Current Allergy Asthma Report. 2018;**18**(10):54